PLAB-2
If You Can, You Can

PLAB-2
If You Can, You Can

This Journey is a Joint Venture of

Soundararajan Sathyan
MBBS   DA   MRSH

Asha Dhandapani
MBBS   MRSH

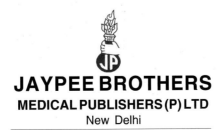

JAYPEE BROTHERS
MEDICAL PUBLISHERS (P) LTD
New Delhi

Published by

Jitendar P Vij

Jaypee Brothers Medical Publishers (P) Ltd

EMCA House, 23/23B Ansari Road, Daryaganj

New Delhi 110 002, India

Phones: +91-11-23272143, +91-11-23272703, +91-11-23282021, +91-11-23245672

Fax: +91-11-23276490, +91-11-23245683   e-mail: jaypee@jaypeebrothers.com

Visit our website: www.jaypeebrothers.com

Branches

- 202 Batavia Chambers, 8 Kumara Krupa Road, Kumara Park East,
  Bangalore 560 001, Phones: +91-80-22285971, +91-80-22382956, +91-80-30614073
  Tele Fax: +91-80-22281761   e-mail: jaypeebc@bgl.vsnl.net.in
- 282 IIIrd Floor, Khaleel Shirazi Estate, Fountain Plaza
  Pantheon Road, **Chennai** 600 008, Phones: +91-44-28262665, +91-44-28269897
  Fax: +91-44-28262331   e-mail: jpmedpub@md3.vsnl.net.in
- 4-2-1067/1-3, lst Floor, Balaji Building, Ramkote
  Cross Road, **Hyderabad** 500 095, Phones: +91-40-55610020, +91-40-24758498
  Fax: +91-40-24758499   e-mail: jpmedpub@rediffmail.com
- 1A Indian Mirror Street, Wellington Square
  Kolkata 700 013, Phone: +91-33-22451926 Fax: +91-33-22456075
  e-mail: jpbcal@cal.vsnl.net.in
- 106 Amit Industrial Estate, 61 Dr SS Rao Road, Near MGM Hospital
  Parel, **Mumbai** 400 012, Phones: +91-22-24124863, +91-22-24104532, +91-22-30926896
  Fax: +91-22-24160828   e-mail: jpmedpub@bom7.vsnl.net.in

PLAB-2 If You Can, You Can

First Edition: 2005

ISBN 81-8061-532-4

Typeset at   JPBMP typesetting unit
Printed at   Paras Offset Pvt. Ltd., C-176, Naraina Ind. Area, New Delhi-28.

Dedicated to
Our loving parents
Dr Soundararajan and Mrs S Subathra
and
Mr M Dhandapani and Mrs D Dhanalakshmi

PLAB-2

Preface

I personally feel that it is not intelligence that is going to help but common sense, presence of mind and communication with body language.

I have gone through the hard-core way in the United Kingdom, and all of this is worth it.

I have dedicated this book to my guide and mentor, my father Dr. N. Soundararajan and my beloved mother Mrs. S. Subathra.

I wish all of you, the very best in PLAB-2 and also for your lives ahead.

Soundararajan Sathyan

PLAB-2 is the next hurdle now after PLAB-1. It was as though I was left in a sea all alone when I thought about PLAB-2 and mannequin especially, as most of us are not exposed to it. But, believe me it is going to be one of the easiest exams that you have faced till date.

All that you need is confidence, good communication skills and you should also be professional.

We have compiled all possible stations here and included a section called *Newer Stations* only to help you.

I dedicate this work to my encouraging and supporting parents, Mr. M. Dhandapani and Mrs. D. Dhanalakshmi who have given me the confidence, the roots of responsibility as well as wings of freedom.

I wish all of them, the very best in PLAB-2 and also a bright future.

Asha Dhandapani

Acknowledgements

No work is complete without due recognition being given to persons who made it possible. Our project is no exception. Many, in their own ways though subtle, influenced it and made a difference for the better. We would like to place on record our profound gratitude for those who have mattered the most in the successful completion of our project.

Firstly, we would like to thank **Mrs. Hemalatha D** for her able guidance from the point of selecting the title till the process of designing the book and helping in getting the counselling cassettes done. Without her help and suggestions for improvement, this project would never have been completed.

We are indebted to **Dr. Veda Murali and Mr. Karthik Dhandapani** for constant encouragement and support.

Our special thanks to Dr. Sivanantha Kumar K. for always being with us, every step of the way.

We are grateful to Mr. Yusuf of PLAB India, Mr. Ganesh, Mr. Audhithan and Mrs. Priya Anand who stood beside us to make the whole project attain a professional stature.

Finally, we would like to thank M/s Jaypee Brothers Medical Publishers (P) Ltd. and especially Mr. R. Jayanandan the author co-ordinator of Chennai branch for his work and all those who have helped us in the completion of this project in their own way.

Contents

PLAB-2

INTRODUCTION

PLAB-2 is a license to work in the United Kingdom. The PLAB-2 exam is an apt one to test our communication skills and our medical knowledge at the same time. These exams are conducted at the level of a house officer and so will not be that difficult as it sounds. At the same time it needs a lot of practice to pass the exams. The doctor-patient relationship is different in the UK when compared to that in our home country. We need to explain everything in detail to the patient; the patient is given a lot of importance there. This aspect being a new concept to us, we need to accustom ourselves to their way and hence this book.

PLAB-2

GENERAL INFORMATION

Eligibility: Pass in PLAB-1

Application: Refer website *www.gmc-uk.org*
The forms can be filled online and fees can be paid through a credit card.

Plab II exam fees: 430 sterling pounds

Exam venue: 1) GMC Venue
178, Great Portland Street
London, W1N 6JE
2) GMC Venue
Clinical Assessment Centre
350 Euston Road
Regents Place
London, NW1 3AX

IN THE EXAMINATION CENTRE

◆ Dress smartly before going.

◆ Always reach the centre at least 30-60 minutes earlier.

◆ Carry all the necessary documents, both original and photocopy which includes the following:

   IELTS Certificate

   PLAB-1 Certificate

   PLAB-2 exams admission ticket

   Passport

   Degree Certificate.

◆ The examination will last for about 96 minutes, 1 hour 36 minutes exactly.

◆ In the centre you will be explained in detail how to proceed and what to do.

ABOUT THE EXAMINATION

You will be taken to a hall and a video clipping will be played which shows how the exams will be carried out.

You will be allotted a particular number between 1-16 and will have to stand outside that room and the next one-minute is for you to read and understand the question. The format of the question is mentioned later.

The next bell you have to enter inside and start off with the station. At 4 minutes and 30 seconds, try to wrap up the station.

The next bell is at 5 minutes and here you will have to leave the room and start reading the next question, as your 1 minute time will be included from the 5 minutes bell.

There are two rest stations or may be one rest station with another one being a pilot station. A pilot station is one, which may be kept for future exams. It is, however, not compulsory to perform the pilot station.

This carries on until for another 16 stations.

At the end you need to collect your belongings and leave the GMC hall.

The results will be announced approximately 15 days later on the net at 12.00 in the noon and will reach you 1 or 2 days later by post.

ADVISE TO ALL CANDIDATES

◆ This exam is at the level of an intern and hence think at that level only.

◆ Prepare at least for one month seriously.

◆ Preparing in a group is always beneficial.

◆ An attachment is not compulsory for a pass but again it is going to be beneficial though I would suggest that it is the practice, which counts now.

◆ "First impression is the best", smile when greeting the examiner, and don't get tensed. Carry on professionally.

◆ No need to change our accent at all.

◆ Do not talk to the examiner or the patient unnecessarily.

◆ The patients will be very co-operative.

◆ Do not use medical terms at all, use layman terms as much as possible.

◆ In case you cannot give an answer, tell him you will refer seniors and let him know.

2 Mock Paper

EXAMINATION PROFILE / MOCK EXAM

There are 16 stations in total. Usually the 8th and 13th station may be rest station. I have mentioned in brief about the 16 stations here.

A CPR station is compulsory for every exam.

History taking	- 2 to 3 stations
Examination	- 2 to 3 stations
Counselling	- 3 to 4 stations
Mannequin	- 2 to 3 stations
CPR	- 1 station
Telephone conversation	- 1 station
Rest stations	- 2 stations

1. URINARY CATHETERIZATION—Procedure

Mr. Harry has come with urinary tract obstruction. Carry on with urinary catheterization.

This is a mannequin station wherein after the general introduction, you need to proceed with cleaning. Doing it sterile way is the main aim of this procedure. As in all mannequins stations explain the entire procedure to the examiner.

2. BREATHLESSNESS—History taking

Mr. Harold was playing football yesterday evening and he had come to Accident and Emergency after having an attack of shortness of breath. Take history from him and arrive at a diagnosis.

Here this is a direct question wherein you need to consider the different diagnosis for breathlessness and take history. It could be CCF; pulmonary edema; asthma; pulmonary embolism; pneumothorax; bronchiectasis

You can consider it as respiratory and CVS causes.

3. ABDOMEN—Examination

Mrs. Kelly has come with pain abdomen, to the Department of Surgery and history has been taken, carry out with the examination.

This is an examination station and with various diagnosis such as acute cholecystitis, acute hepatitis, gastritis, renal causes, appendicitis, cystitis, ectopic pregnancy, PID; you need to carry on with the examination in the order of inspection, palpation, percussion and auscultation.

4. DEPRESSION—Counselling

A 26 years old Mr. Richter had come to the psychiatry clinic with depression and you the Senior House Officer in the Department have to discuss about TCA, his medication.

Here the diagnosis being already made, you need to discuss about the antidepressant and its action, the side effects, you also have to advise him about his driving and to follow the prescription regularly.

5. CRANIAL NERVE II-VII — Examination

Examine II- VII Cranial nerve while explaining all your findings to the examiner.

There is a person (simulator) here with intact cranial nerve but may act as if he is having some deficit, explain the procedure to the patient and also the examiner. Here the examiner will note how fluent you are with carrying the procedure and whether you are performing it the right way.

6. HOT FLUSHES AND SWEATS—History and Counselling

Mrs. Winston has come to the gynecology clinic with mood swings and night sweats and hot flushes. She is 35 years old. Take history and counsel her.

Here the diagnosis is evident to be premature menopause, it is your work to elicit a history of menopause with all the symptoms and to rule out the cause, which could be premature menopause, any surgery involving the ovary or uterus, radiological procedure, if it runs in family, tuberculosis, chemotherapy. Then you have to talk to her in brief about menopause and the treatment modalities available.

7. PERFORM CPR—Basic Life Support

There is a male patient found collapsed in the cubicle, perform CPR.

This is a compulsory station wherein you have to perform BLS. Here the examiner will note your skill in resuscitation. A pass in all the stations but a blunder in this can prove to be very costly.

8. REST STATION

You can rest here for totally 6 minutes.

9. WHEEZE—History Taking

Miss Freeman has come to the Accident and Emergency with wheeze; you are the SHO there. Elicit a detailed history and come to a diagnosis.

This station tests your history taking skills and here the diagnosis could be asthma, bronchiectasis, pneumonia, pleural effusion, (RS causes) and CCF, MI, pulmonary embolism (CVS causes), anemia, hysterical.

You should be able to come to a diagnosis at the end.

10. TELEPHONE CONVERSATION

You are the SHO on call in Surgery and the nurse calls you to the ward to examine a patient who had undergone herniorrhaphy 8 hours back. His vitals are mentioned in the chart and on examination his tummy is distended.

Converse with the Consultant, Mr. Reaper about this.

This can be one of the stations in PLAB-2 wherein the examiner, i.e. the consultant on call will be sitting on other side of the screen and a chart placed in front of you with a telephone beside. Here the examiner will test how well you can inform the situation and how good you are at managing an emergency like this one.

11. SPACER DEVICE

Mrs. Jones has come with her little one, who is diagnosed as having asthma and you being the Pediatric SHO explain her about it and answer all her queries.

This tests your ability to explain about a common and simple device. Here it is necessary to explain regarding the device to the patient and its advantage and disadvantage as well. Also you have to explain the cleaning aspects. The ultimate aim here is to make the patient understand every thing about the device.

12. BLOOD PRESSURE MEASUREMENT

Measure the blood pressure of this patient who has come to you with dizziness. Do not take history.

This is a straightforward question wherein you need to measure blood pressure both, by palpatory and auscultatory method. Also we need to check the BP in both sitting and standing position. Do not forget to note the values.

13. REST STATION

14. OPHTHALMOSCOPY

Perform ophthalmoscopic examination on the mannequin and give a description of the fundus.

This is another mannequin station. Address the mannequin indirectly and don't forget to do the general examination of the eye before the actual procedure.

15. BREAKING BAD NEWS—Counselling

Following examining Mrs. Gibbs and running few tests it was diagnosed that she has cancer of the right breast and it is in an advanced stage now. Break this news to her.

Here it is necessary to get into the situation and then break the news gently taking care of the patient's sensitivity.

It is very important to be frank and to tell about the exact diagnosis to the patient.

Give a pause wherever necessary and later tell her what can be done to make her feel better. Never give any false assurances to any one.

16. OBTAINING CONSENT FOR HERNIORRHAPHY—Counselling

Mr. Pick has come with right inguinal hernia and after consultation, Herniorrhaphy was suggested. Obtain consent for the procedure.

This is a very common station and its explanation is with defining hernia to the patient and then to tell him the need of the surgery, the side effect, the postoperative care.

At the end of the session provide him with the consent form and get it signed after he is satisfied.

3 General Introduction and Common Terms

The OSCE'S are conducted at the level of a medical graduate. All these stations are those, which we have practiced during our medical career. It is this knowledge along with confidence that has to be used in combination during the exams.

In all these stations, it is necessary to listen to what the patient (simulators) have got to say. Believe me, it is they who will lead to our success in PLAB-2. You need to request, appreciate, congratulate, thank and explain things to the patient. Whatever you do in the PLAB-2 exams is what you do in the NHS in the UK. An attachment will definitely help you for your exam but, however, it is not compulsory.

HISTORY TAKING

Here, it is necessary to elicit history about a particular condition. The patient will lead you to the diagnosis.

COUNSELLING

It is necessary to understand the question/situation before counselling. We also do this in our hospitals, but the conversation is usually one-way. In OSCE and NHS, it is an important part to have counselling done and in as a two-way conversation. Allow the patients to ask questions. This decides our success too.

MANNEQUIN

Here we do those procedures, which we have already performed as house-surgeons (PRHO/HO). It is important to keep talking to the examiner or the mannequin as indicated.

BASIC SKILLS

There are no excuses for not knowing these and most importantly in exact steps. We are not aware of primary and secondary survey. Here, we have given a detailed description of all basic skills, which is what the GMC and NHS expect. This holds an important part of the exams.

CLINICAL EXAMINATION

These are simple and easy to perform and also to complete it within the said 5 minutes that GMC provides. We have practiced these umpteen number of times. So, no worries about this part.

TELEPHONE CONVERSATION

Usually, they may have one of this station wherein they test how well and how specific and accurate we are when we call our senior to see a patient.

VIVA STATIONS

This is in a way something like the viva we face during our exams in Medical school. We have to be thorough with a few topics from the OHCM – Emergencies.

NOTE:

Always remember that the examiners are never tough nor are the patients unfriendly. They do help us to go through the station successfully.

We have included a new section called *NEW STATIONS*. This, we believe, will be of immense help to all of you as it contains the unusual stations, which have been asked.

Here is a list of few common medical terms, which are in common use in the UK along with the laymen terms.

ORGANS

Medical Terms		*Layman Terms*
Abdomen	-	Tummy
Umbilicus	-	Belly button
Vagina	-	Front passage
Anus/rectum	-	Back passage

Uterus	-	Womb
Cervix	-	Neck of womb
Ovary	-	Egg producing gland
Urinary bladder	-	Water bag
Urethra	-	Water pipe
Prostate	-	Gland at the neck of water bag
Lymph nodes	-	Gland
Trachea	-	Windpipe
Esophagus	-	Food pipe
Intestine	-	Bowel
Retina	-	Back of eye

COMMON TERMS

Nausea	-	Feeling sick
Vomiting	-	Sickness
Diarrhea (Diarrhoea)	-	Runs
Urine	-	Pee/water
Urine passage	-	Water works
Passing stools	-	Opening bowel/poo
Stools	-	Waste
Tablets	-	Medicine
Drugs	-	Recreational drugs
Incision	-	Nick
Pfannensteil incision	-	Bikini line nick
Fever	-	Running temperature
Anaesthetize	-	Put to sleep
OCP	-	Pills
Analgesics	-	Pain killers
Diuretic	-	Water tablet
Stool softener	-	Laxative
Anticoagulant	-	Blood thinners
Radiotherapy	-	Strong X-ray therapy
USG	-	TV scan

PLAB-2

ECG	-	Trace of heart
EEG	-	Trace of brain
CTG	-	Trace of baby
Vaccination	-	Jabs
IUCD	-	Coil
Microorganisms	-	Bugs

PLAB-2

4 *History Taking*

HISTORY TAKING

This section tests our ability to diagnose an illness and to rule out the others. Introduction should always be perfect. It is the first part and most important part of any station. This will create a very good impression and will help you to take the patient into confidence. Further, the station would go on smooth. There is a standard pattern to be followed in history taking.

◆ Introduction: This includes greeting the patient, introducing yourself, checking the identity, building a rapport, explaining the purpose of your visit.
(GIIRP: GREET, INTRODUCE, IDENTITY, RAPPORT, PURPOSE)

◆ Ask questions pertaining to the complaint (E.g: In case of chest pain, ask everything about the pain – the site, onset, duration, aggravating and relieving factors, nature and radiation).

◆ Ask questions to find the diagnosis and to rule out the differential diagnosis.

◆ Past history.

◆ Personal history including history of smoking, drinking and use of recreational drugs.

◆ Family history.

◆ Medication history

◆ Allergy history.

◆ Conclusion.

By now you would have completed the station and that too covering all the important points.

DIFFERENTIAL DIAGNOSIS FOR HISTORY TAKING

1. **CHEST PAIN**
    - ◆ Angina
    - ◆ Myocardial infarction
    - ◆ Pulmonary embolism _acute dyspnea, pleuritic chest pain, hemoptosis, syncope, pleural rub_
    - ◆ GERD _heartburn, regurgitation of acid or bile, excessive salivation, odynophagia (severe esophagitis or stricture), nocturnal asthma (wheeze or cough)_
    - ◆ Pleurisy
    - ◆ Trauma

2. **PALPITATION**
    - ◆ SVT/VT/MI
    - ◆ Anxiety/Panic attacks
    - ◆ Thyrotoxicosis
    - ◆ Phaeochromocytoma
    - ◆ Hypoglycaemia
    - ◆ Excess coffee
    - ◆ Stress
    - ◆ Drugs/Medication

3. **WHEEZE**
    - ◆ Asthma
    - ◆ Pneumonia
    - ◆ MI/CCF
    - ◆ Pulmonary embolism
    - ◆ Pulmonary edema

4. **BREATHLESSNESS**
    - ◆ Asthma
    - ◆ Pneumonia
    - ◆ Bronchiectasis
    - ◆ Pleural effusion
    - ◆ Cancer lung
    - ◆ MI/CCF
    - ◆ Pulmonary edema/embolism
    - ◆ Anaemia

5. **LOSS OF WEIGHT**
    ◆ Cancer
    ◆ Tuberculosis
    ◆ Anorexia nervosa
    ◆ Hyperthyroidism
    ◆ Diabetes mellitus
    ◆ MAS *(malabsorption syndrome)*
    ◆ IBS
    ◆ Depression
    ◆ Drugs

6. **CONSTIPATION**
    ◆ Colorectal cancer
    ◆ IBD
    ◆ IBS
    ◆ Intestinal obstruction
    ◆ Anal fissure
    ◆ Functional
    ◆ Sedentary
    ◆ Old age
    ◆ Depression
    ◆ Drugs/Medication ① opiate analgesics eg morphine, codein, ② anticholinergics eg tricyclics, phenothiazines, ③ iron

7. **DIARRHOEA**
    ◆ Acute gastroenteritis
    ◆ Food poisoning
    ◆ Cancer colon
    ◆ IBD
    ◆ IBS
    ◆ MAS
    ◆ Hyperthyroidism
    ◆ Pseudomembranous colitis
    ◆ Drugs/Medication - laxative abuse, antibiotics, cimetidine, propranolol, cytotoxics, digoxin, alcohol.

8. **HEADACHE**
    ◆ Migraine
    ◆ Subarachnoid haemorrhage

◆ Epilepsy

◆ Meningitis/Encephalitis

◆ Glaucoma/Refractive error

◆ Giant cell arteritis

◆ Tension headache/cluster headache

◆ Sinusitis

◆ ICSOL   intra cranial space occupying lesion.

◆ Trauma

◆ Malaria

9. **LOSS OF CONSCIOUSNESS**

◆ Epilepsy

◆ Meningitis

◆ Encephalitis

◆ Diabetes/Hypoglycaemia

◆ Drop attack*— no loss of consciousness, only sudden weakness of legs

◆ Stokes-Adams attack/SVT/VT

◆ Vasovagal attack

◆ Carotid sinus syndrome

◆ Drugs/Medications

◆ Anxiety/Hysterical

◆ ICSOL

10. **VOMITING**

◆ Acute gastroenteritis

◆ Food poisoning

◆ Migraine

◆ Meningitis

◆ Encephalitis

◆ Glaucoma

◆ Refractive error

◆ ICSOL

◆ Pregnancy

◆ Intestinal obstruction

◆ Acute appendicitis

◆ Acute cholecystitis

11. **DYSPHAGIA**
    ◆ Cancer oesophagus
    ◆ Cancer pharynx
    ◆ Pharyngeal pouch
    ◆ Globus hystericus
    ◆ Plummer-Vinson syndrome
    ◆ GERD/Achalasia

12. **PAIN ABDOMEN**
    ◆ Acute cholecystitis
    ◆ Hepatitis
    ◆ Pneumonia
    ◆ Kidney stone
    ◆ UTI
    ◆ Duodenal ulcer
    ◆ Gastritis
    ◆ PID
    ◆ Ectopic pregnancy
    ◆ Salpingitis
    ◆ Appendicitis
    ◆ Cystitis
    ◆ Urinary tract obstruction

13. **URINARY TRACT OBSTRUCTION**
    ◆ Cancer prostate
    ◆ Prostatitis
    ◆ BPH
    ◆ Cancer bladder
    ◆ Kidney stone
    ◆ Urethral stricture
    ◆ Trauma

14. **BLEEDING PER RECTUM**
    ◆ Cancer colon
    ◆ Haemorroid
    ◆ Anal fissure
    ◆ IBD

◆ Amoebic dysentery

◆ Trauma

◆ Rectal prolapse

◆ Colonic polyp/Diverticulosis

◆ Bleeding diathesis

15. HAEMATURIA T₁ -diathermy via cystoscope (intravesical chemotherapeutic agents for multiple small tumor. T2-3 - cystectomy + chemotherapy + irradiation.

◆ Cancer bladder T₄ - palliative radiotherapy, urinary diversion to ↓ pain.

nocturia, hesitancy, poor stream, terminal dribbling or urinary obstruction.

◆ Cancer prostate - nerve sparing radical prostectomy, radiotherapy. Hormones : GnRH eg goserelin Zoladex Sc.

◆ Prostatitis

◆ UTI (Cystitis) - Frequency, dysuria, urgency, strangury, haematuria, suprapubic pain.
→ drink plenty of fluids, void after intercourse, trimethoprim 12hr/200mg PO 3days.

◆ Kidney stone - <5mm, no intervention unless obstructn or infectn. <2cm Lithotripsy. Renal colic: IV fluids, diclofenac, morphine + metoclopramid, antibiotics, retrograde stent insertion, nephrostomy. (urology refer)

◆ Schistosomiasis (africa, middle east, Indian Ocean) → frequency, dysuria, hematuria, incontinnue Praziquantel 40mg/kg PO with food in 2 doses.

◆ Gonorrhoea

◆ Bleeding diathesis

16. AMENORRHOEA

◆ Physiological

◆ Late starter

◆ Imperforate hymen

◆ Anorexia nervosa

◆ Pregnancy

◆ Tuberculosis

◆ PCOD

◆ Pituitary tumour

◆ Premature menopause

◆ Menopause

◆ Pills

17. BLEEDING PER VAGINUM

◆ Abortion

◆ Ectopic pregnancy

◆ Fibroid

◆ Endometriosis

◆ PID

- Cervicitis
- Trauma
- Cancer cervix
- Cancer endometrium

18. **CHILD WITH FEVER**
    - Meningitis/Encephalitis
    - UTI
    - Diabetes mellitus
    - GIT upset
    - Otitis media/upper respiratory tract infection
    - Sinusitis
    - Febrile convulsion

19. **CRYING CHILD**
    - Intussusception
    - UTI
    - GERD
    - Ear pain

20. **FEBRILE CONVULSION**

21. **DIABETIC CHILD**
    - Diabetes mellitus
    - Diabetes insipidus
    - ICSOL
    - UTI
    - Head injury

22. **UTI IN CHILD**

23. **DIARRHOEA IN CHILD**

24. **DEPRESSION**

25. **POSTNATAL DEPRESSION**

26. **POST-TRAUMATIC STRESS DISORDER**

27. **ALCOHOL HISTORY**

28. **CHILD ABUSE**

29. **ANOREXIA NERVOSA (Same as Station 5)**

PLAB-2

PLAB-2

MEDICINE

1. CHEST PAIN

Mr. Freeman, a 45-years old businessman was playing football when he suddenly suffered from chest pain and was brought to casualty. Take relevant history from him. You are SHO in accident and emergency.

Good Morning Mr. Freeman. How are you? I am Dr. ABC, Senior House Officer in Accident and Emergency, as far as I know you have come here with chest discomfort. I would like to ask you a few questions regarding this to find out what is causing this. Is that all right? Are you comfortable?

◆ Where did the pain first show?

   When did it start?

   Can you describe the pain for me?

   Does it spread anywhere else?

   What makes it worse?

   What makes you feel better? Is it increasing further?

◆ Do you feel suffocated during this period and sweat excessively? **(Angina; MI)**

◆ Did you travel on air recently?

   Did you have pain in your leg?

   Did you undergo any surgery recently or were you admitted for long in hospital?

   (Pulmonary embolism)

◆ Did you feel sourness in the mouth?

   Is this pain related to your food intake? **(GERD)**

   Does the pain increase while bending forward or lying down?

◆ Did you sustain trauma to the chest? **(Trauma)**

◆ Did you have running temperature, cough with phlegm? **(Pleurisy)**

◆ Did you have similar experience in the past?

   Any other illness or any surgeries?

   Have you had a stroke or a heart attack?

   Have you had any other heart problems?

◆ Do you smoke? Do you drink? Do you use any recreational drugs?

◆ Do you have high blood pressure or high blood sugar?

◆ Did anyone else have similar problems in your family?

Does anyone in your family have high blood pressure, stroke or any heart problem?

Did anyone have sudden death in your family?

◆ Are you on any medication?

◆ Are you allergic to anything?

✔ Is there anything else that you would like to tell me?

I appreciate your co-operation. I'll come back to you later.

Don't worry; we'll take care of you.

Thanks.

2. PALPITATION

Miss Jamal has come with excess pounding of the heart. She is 17 years old and worried and also anxious about something serious that might have happened. Take a relevant history from her.

Good Morning Miss. Jamal. How are you feeling today? I am Dr. ABC, Senior House Officer in Medicine. I am here to ask you about the problem with which you are here. Is that OK? Are you comfortable?

◆ When did you notice this excess pounding of the heart?

How did it start?

Is it present all the time or occasionally?

Does anything worsen it?

What makes you feel better?

Is it regular?

How long does it last?

◆ Do you have chest pain, difficulty in breathing, suffocating sensation or excess sweating? **(SVT; VT; MI)**

◆ Do you dislike heat? Do you feel you have lost weight? What about your bowel habits? **(Thyrotoxicosis)**

◆ Do you feel suffocated amidst crowds, in market place?   agoraphobia

Do you feel tensed especially about the future and feel something bad is going to happen? **(Panic attacks)**

◆ Do you feel dizzy or tired? Do you pee frequently? **(Hypoglycaemia)**

◆ Do you get frequent headaches, running temperature, shaking of hands? **(Phaeochromocytoma)**

Have you had similar experience in the past? Any other illness or any surgeries in the past?

Have you had stroke? Any heart problem?

◆ Do you smoke, drink or use any recreational drugs? Do you have high blood pressure or high blood sugar?

◆ Are you worried about any exams, job, and family?

◆ Anyone in your family with similar problems?

◆ Are you on any medication? Are you allergic to anything?

Is there anything else that you would like to tell me?

I appreciate your co-operation. Don't worry; we'll take care of you.

Thank you.

3. WHEEZE

Mr. Jason has been complaining of wheeze since a couple of hours. He has come to A+E, you being the SHO on call take a relevant history from him and discuss the diagnosis with the examiner.

Good Morning Mr. Jason, I am Dr. ABC, Senior House Officer in Accident and Emergency, How are you feeling? Are you comfortable? As far as I know, you have come here with wheeze. I would like to ask you a few questions regarding this so that we can find out what's causing it? Is that OK?

◆ When did it start?

How did the wheeze start?

What worsens this?

What makes you feel better?

Is it present all the time or occasionally? Is it present when you lie down?

Is it more in the early mornings?

◆ Do you have itching eyes and nose, red eye and running nose?

Does it get aggravated when you are in garden?

Did you change your house or job recently?

Does the problem increase when you are with your pets?

Did you enter into a cleaning spree recently?

Did you eat any food-causing allergy? **(Asthma)**

◆ Do you have running temperature, cough, phlegm? **(Pneumonia)**
◆ Do you have chest pain, suffocation, and difficulty in breathing? **(MI, pulmonary oedema, CCF)**
◆ Did you travel on air recently?

Do you have pain in the leg?

Did you undergo any surgery recently? **(Pulmonary embolism)**
◆ Were you diagnosed as having asthma, hay fever, eczema or any other allergy?

Have you had similar experience in the past?
◆ Do you smoke, drink or use any drugs?

Do you have high blood pressure or high blood sugar?
◆ Does anyone else in your family have similar experience? Anyone with asthma, hay fever?
◆ Are you on any medication? Are you allergic to anything?

Is there anything else that you would like to tell?

I appreciate your co-operation.

Don't worry we're here to take care of you. I'll come back to you later. Thank You. Bye.

4. BREATHLESSNESS

Mr. Lewensky is 56 years old working in the bank. He has come to the A+E after an attack of shortness of breath. Take history from him.

Hello Mr. Lewensky, I am Dr. ABC, Senior House Officer in Accident and Emergency, How are you feeling? I am here to ask you a few questions regarding your problem. We'll get to know what's causing this and can treat you early. Is that OK with you?
◆ Since when are you finding it difficult to breathe?

How did it start?

What worsens the condition? What makes you feel better?

Is it present all the time or occasionally?

Does this problem arise as soon as you lie down or following 2-3 hours after sleep?
◆ Did you have chest pain with suffocation and excess sweating? Does your heart pound excessively? **(MI, pulmonary oedema, CCF)**

◆ Do you get it only when you are amidst crowds or in market place? **(Anxiety, panic attacks)**

◆ Do you have this problem when you are cleaning the house, with your pet, gardening? **(Asthma)**

◆ Do you have running temperature, cough and phlegm?**(Bronchiectasis, pneumonia)**

◆ Did you travel on air recently?

Did you undergo any surgery or were you hospitalised recently for long?

Do you have pain in the leg? **(Pulmonary embolism)**

◆ Do you feel you have lost your weight and appetite?

Have you noticed any glands in your body? **(Cancer lung)**

◆ Have you had similar experience in the past? Any surgeries, any medical illness?

Were you diagnosed as having hay fever, asthma?

Do you have any other heart problem?

◆ Do you smoke? Do you drink or use any drugs? Do you have a high blood pressure or high blood sugar?

◆ Are you on any medication?

◆ Are you allergic to anything?

◆ Does anyone else in your family have similar experience?

Is there anything else that you would like to tell me? Thanks for your co-operation.

Don't worry; we'll take care of you. Thank You.

5. WEIGHT LOSS

Miss Andrea, 16 years old girl has been brought to the hospital by her mother with complaints of losing weight. Take relevant history.

Hello Miss. Andrea? I am Dr. ABC, Senior House Officer in Medicine. How are you feeling? I am here to have small talk with you. Is that OK?

◆ What did you have for breakfast?

Did you sleep well?

◆ What do you feel about your weight?

Can you tell me what your previous weight was? What is it now? In how many days have you lost this weight?

What do your family and friends comment about your weight?

How many hours do you spend in the Gym?

Can you tell me your diet schedule?

Do you take laxatives or induce sickness?

What type of clothes do you prefer wearing?

Who is your role model?

Do you feel energetic to do your work?

Have you had any thoughts or idea of harming yourself?

What do you feel the future has in store for you?

Are you interested in social gathering, parties and shopping? **(Anorexia nervosa)**

◆ Have you lost your appetite? Did you notice any glands in your body? **(Cancer)**

◆ What about your bowel habits?

Does the waste float in water? **(MAS)**

◆ Did you travel to any Asian country? Do you have cough, running temperature?

Did you come in contact wit anyone with tuberculosis? **(Tuberculosis)**

◆ Do you dislike heat? **(Thyrotoxicosis)**

◆ Do you feel low? Do you dislike the future? **(Depression)**

◆ Can I ask you something personal?

Are you worried about your family?

Worried about your job, finance?

What about your periods and your sexual life?

◆ Did you donate blood or receive blood recently or got yourself tattooed? **(Hepatitis)**

◆ Do you pee frequently and feel more thirsty? **(Diabetes)**

◆ Have you had similar experience in the past? Do you have any other illness?

◆ Do you smoke or drink? Do you use any recreational drugs? Do you have high blood pressure or high blood sugar?

◆ Does anyone else have similar experience in your family? Anyone with tuberculosis, cancer?

◆ Are you on any medication? Are you allergic to anything?

Is there anything else that you would like to tell me?

You have been very co-operative.

I'll come back to you later. Take care. Thanks

PLAB-2

6. CONSTIPATION

Mr. Francis is here after undergoing herniorrhaphy. He is complaining of difficulty in opening the bowel. Take history and come to a diagnosis.

Hello Mr. Francis. I am Dr. ABC, Senior House Officer in Medicine. How are you feeling today? I am here to ask you a few questions regarding your complaint so that we can find out what is causing it. Is it ok ?

- Since when are you having this problem?
  Once in how many days do you open your bowel?
  What worsens this condition?
  What makes you feel better?
  Is there any bleeding from the back passage?
- Have you lost your weight recently? What about your appetite? Did you notice any glands in your body?
  Does this problem alternate with runs? **(Cancer colon)**
- Do you have pain in the back passage? **(Anal fissure)**
- Do you have any rashes on your body, any joint pain, and red eye? **(IBD)**
- Do you have pain in the tummy? Did you pass wind? Do you have sickness? **(Intestinal obstruction)**
- Do you feel low? Do you feel worthless, hopeless? Have you lost your sleep? **(Depression)**
- Were you hospitalised recently? Did you change your job or house recently? **(Functional)**
- Do you dislike cold? Do you feel you have put on weight? **(Hypothyroidism)**
- Are you on any medications like morphine?
- Have you had similar problems in the past? Any other medical illness? Any surgeries?
- Do you smoke, drink or use any recreational drugs? Do you have high blood pressure or high blood sugar?
- Anyone in your family with similar problems?
- Are you on any medication or allergic to anything?
  Anything else you would like to tell?
  You have been very co-operative. Thank you. I'll come back to you again. Bye.

PLAB-2

7. DIARRHOEA

Here is Mr. Alexander, who is been troubled by runs. You are the SHO in Medicine. Take history from him.

Hello Mr. Alexander. I am Dr. XYZ, Senior House Officer in Medicine. How are you feeling? As far as I know you have come here with runs. I would like to ask you a few questions regarding this to find out what's causing it. Is that OK?

◆ Since when are you having runs?

How many times in a day do you poo?

Does anything worsen it? What makes you feel better?

Is it watery or semi-solid?

Does it contain blood in it?

Does it have a bad smell?

Do you find difficulty to flush the waste? **(MAS)**

◆ Do you have to poo as soon as you wake up?

Do you have problems with opening your bowel alternately? Have you lost weight and appetite recently? Did you notice any glands in your body? **(Cancer colon)**

◆ Do you have temperature?

Do you have pain in the tummy? Do you feel sick? **(Acute gastroenteritis)**

◆ Does anyone else have similar problems in your family? Did you have food elsewhere? Did you travel out recently? **(Food poisoning)**

◆ Do you dislike heat? **(Thyrotoxicosis)**

◆ Are you on any medications or laxatives? **(Pseudomembraneous colitis; laxative abuse)**

◆ Do you have any joint pain, red eye? **(IBD)**

◆ Did you have similar experience in the past? Any other medical illness?

◆ Do you smoke, drink or use any recreational drugs? Do you have high blood pressure and high blood sugar?

◆ Anyone in your family with similar problems?

◆ Are you on any medication or allergic to anything?

Anything else you would like to tell?

You have been very co-operative. Thank you. I'll come back to you again. Bye.

8. HEADACHE

Mrs. Friedman has been suffering with headache since few hours. Obtain a relevant history from her regarding this.

Hello Mrs. Friedman, how are you feeling today? I am Dr. XYZ, Senior House Officer in Medicine. I am here to ask you few questions regarding your problems, so that we can find out what is causing it. Are you comfortable?

♦ Where is the pain?

   Since when are you having it?

   Did it start all of a sudden?

   Does the pain go anywhere else?

   Can you describe the pain?

   What worsens it? What makes you feel better?

   Does this pain come from elsewhere?

♦ Do you feel this, as the worst headache in your life? –

   Do you feel as if someone has knocked you on the back of your head? **(SAH)**

♦ Do you have running temperature? Do you avoid light? Do you feel sick? Do you have stiffness in the neck? **(Meningitis, encephalitis)**

♦ Did you have fits?   **(Epilepsy)**

♦ Did you have a premonition prior to this attack? Did you notice any zigzag spots in front of your eyes? **(Migraine)**

♦ Do you have running temperature or running nose? Any cold or cough? **(Sinusitis)**

♦ Do you see haloes around light? **(Glaucoma)**

♦ Do you have any problem with your vision?

♦ Do you get this headache once in a month? Does your eye get swollen and become red? Is it more in the night? **(Cluster headache)**

♦ Are you stressed or worried which increases the headache? Do you feel a tight band around your head? **(Tension headache)**

♦ Do you get it in early morning hours with sickness and fits? **(ICSOL)** Intracranial space occupying lesion.

♦ Did you travel to other countries recently? **(Malaria)**

♦ Have you had similar experience in the past? Any other medical, surgical or psychiatric illness?

♦ Do you smoke, drink, use any recreational drugs?

♦ Do you have a high blood pressure or a high blood sugar?

◆ Anyone in your family with similar experience? Anyone with migraine or ICSOL?

◆ Are you on any medication? Are you allergic to anything?

Anything else that you would like to tell me?

I appreciate your co-operation. Thanks I'll come back to you again. Bye.

9. LOSS OF CONSCIOUSNESS

Mr. Brandon, 45 years old teacher had lost his consciousness, he is now in the Medicine OPD. Take relevant history from him.

Good Morning Mr. Brandon, how are you? I am Dr. XYZ, Senior House Officer in Medicine. As far as I know you had come with complaints of loss of consciousness. I am here to ask you a few questions regarding it so that we can find out what's causing it. Is that ok? Are you comfortable?

◆ Can you describe what happened?

When did it occur?

What were you doing – exercising, working?

Is this the first time?

How long did it last?

Was there any witness?

◆ Did you have a headache prior to the attack?

Did you have jerking of hands and legs?

Did you bite your tongue? Did you pee during the attack? Did you open bowel during the act?

Did you feel drowsy after the attack? **(Epilepsy)**

◆ Did you have running temperature, headache?

Any neck stiffness or rash on your body? **(Meningitis/Encephalitis)**

◆ Do you pee frequently? Do you feel you have lost weight or put on more? **(Diabetes)**

◆ Are you stressed up a lot? Do you feel suffocated in crowds? Do you loose your consciousness in crowds or in particular situations? **(Panic attack, anxiety)**

◆ Does this occur when you are shaving or massaging your neck? **(Carotid sinus syndrome)**

◆ Do you have chest pain or excess pounding of the heart? **(Stokes-Adams syndrome)**

- Have you had similar experience in the past?
- Do you smoke? Do you drink or use drugs?
- What about your blood sugar and blood pressure?
- Anyone in your family with similar problems, any heart problems, stroke?
- Are you on any medication? Are you allergic to anything?

  Is there anything else that you would like to tell me?

  You have been very co-operative, I appreciate that. I will come back to you later. Thanks.

10. VOMITING

Mrs. Jennifer is admitted in the A+E with sickness. You being the SHO there, take appropriate history from her.

Good Morning Mrs. Jennifer. I am Dr. ABC, Senior House Officer in Accident and Emergency. How are you feeling? As far as I know you have come here with sickness? I would like to ask you a few questions regarding this so that we can find out what is causing it. Is that OK?

- When did it start?

  Is it only sickness or do you feel sick?

  Did it start suddenly?

  How many times did you have sickness?

  What was the color of contents? What were the contents?

  Do you feel sick immediately after eating?

  Does anything worsen it? What makes you feel better?

  Do you feel very tired; do you feel thirsty and pee less?

- Do you have running temperature and runs? Do you have pain in the tummy? **(Acute gastroenteritis)**
- Do you have headache? Do you feel zig-zag designs in front of your eye? **(Migraine)**
- Do you have running temperature? Any neck stiffness? Did you have fits? **(Meningitis, encephalitis)**
- Do you have problems with your vision? **(Refractive error)**
- Could you be pregnant? Are you on pills? **(Pregnancy)**
- Did you open your bowel? Did you pass wind? **(Intestinal obstruction)**
- Have you had similar such episodes previously? Any other medical illness or surgeries that you have undergone?

◆ Do you smoke? Do you drink or use drugs?

◆ What about your blood sugar and blood pressure?

◆ Are you on any medication? Are you allergic to anything that you know?

   Is there anything else that you would like to tell me?

   You have been very co-operative, I appreciate that. Take care and thanks.
   I will come back to you later.

11. DYSPHAGIA

Mr. Richard, 65 years old has come with complaints of difficulty in swallowing since few days. Speak to him and ask about it to find the cause.

Hello Mr. Richard, how are you feeling? I am Dr. XYZ, Senior House Officer in Medicine. I am here to ask you a few questions regarding your complaints so that we can find out what is causing it.

◆ When did you first notice this problem? Was it sudden or building up since a few days?

   What worsens it? What makes you feel better?

   Is it present all the time?

   Is it for only solid or liquid or for both?

◆ Have you noticed any changes in your weight?

   What about your food habits? Did you notice any glands in your body? **(Cancer esophagus/Pharynx)**

◆ Does the food stick in the throat? **(Cancer pharynx)**

◆ Does it seem to occur after taking spicy food or when lying down? **(GERD, achalasia)**

◆ Have you noticed any lump or swelling in the neck? Do you have any bad breath? **(Pharyngeal pouch)**

◆ Do you find suffocating amidst crowd and in market place, excess pounding of the heart, dry mouth?

   Do you feel that food gets stuck in your throat especially at particular situations? **(Globus hystericus)**

◆ Do you feel tired, lethargic with painful lesions at the corner of the mouth? **(Plummer-Vinson syndrome)** *Patterson - Brown - kelly Syndrome.*

◆ Have you had similar experience previously? Any other medical illness or surgeries?

◆ Do you smoke? Do you drink or use drugs?

◆ What about your blood sugar and blood pressure?

◆ Anyone in your family with similar problems, any one with cancer of food pipe or throat?

◆ Are you on any medication? Are you allergic to anything?

   Is there anything else that you would like to tell me?

   You have been very co-operative, I appreciate that. Thanks.

12. PAIN ABDOMEN

Mrs. Jane, 45 years old mother of three children, has come with pain in the tummy since few hours. You are the SHO in surgery. Take relevant history.

Good Morning Mrs. Jane, how are you feeling? I am Dr. ABC, Senior House Officer in Surgery. As far as I know you have come with pain in the tummy. I would like to ask you few questions regarding this so that we can find out what is causing it.

◆ Where is the pain exactly?

   When did it start? Can you describe the pain?

   Does it go elsewhere?

   What worsens it? What makes you feel better?

   Is it present continuously or occasionally?

◆ Do you have sickness? Does the pain increase after taking fatty food? **(Acute Cholecystitis)**

◆ Did you travel to foreign places recently, receive blood or donate? Did you get yourself tattooed? **(Hepatitis)**

◆ Do you have cough, any phlegm? Does this pain increase when breathing? **(Pneumonia)**

◆ Do you have running temperature? Any problem with waterworks? **(Renal causes-UTI)**

◆ Could you be pregnant? Are you on pills? Do you have any bleeding from front passage? **(Ectopic pregnancy)**

◆ Do you have runs? **(Gastroenteritis)**

◆ Have you had similar experience in the past? Any other medical illness or surgeries?

◆ Do you smoke? Do you drink or use drugs?

◆ What about your blood sugar and blood pressure?

◆ Anyone in your family with similar problems?

◆ Are you on any medication? Are you allergic to anything?

Is there anything else that you would like to tell me?

You have been very co-operative; I'll come back to you later. Thanks.

Post operative advice
1) No driving 2w postop
2) 2w no sex
3) 2w bid in urine.
4) If ↑ temp or urinating is painful, bring a sample of urine.

SURGERY

TURP
Pre-op consent on risk
1 - haematuria
2 - hematospermia
3 - hypothermia
4 - Urethral trauma/strictures
5 - Post TURP syndrom (↓T, ↓Na⁺)

6 - Infection, Prostahhs
7 - Impotence
8 - Incontinence
9 - clot retention near stricture
10 - Retrograde ejaculation

13. URINARY TRACT OBSTRUCTION

Mr. Altmann is in the surgery OPD with complaints of not passing water since two days. Obtain history from him.

Hello Mr. Altmann, how are you feeling? I am Dr. XYZ, Senior House Officer in Surgery. I am here to ask you a few questions regarding your complaint so that we can find out what is causing it. Is that ok with you?

◆ When did you first notice this problem?

Was it sudden or building up gradually?

What worsens it? What makes you feel better?

◆ Do you have painful waterworks?

Do you have difficulty in peeing? urinating.

Do you have to rush to the toilet?

Do you have to wait for some time in the loo before you can pee? (hesitancy) BPH

Do you empty your water bag fully?

Do you pee frequently? Does the flow stop start? do you go on dribbling even after a good shake? (terminal dribbling) BPH

Do you leak water when coughing/straining? **(Prostate hypertrophy)**

◆ Do you have running temperature? Have you noticed any white threads/discharge from the water pipe? **(Prostatis, gonorrhoea)**

◆ Do you feel you have lost your weight? What about your appetite? Have you noticed any glands in your body?

Did you notice blood in the water? **(Cancer prostate, cancer bladder)**

◆ Do you have pain in the tummy? Did you pass any stone in your waterwork?

(Urinary stones)

◆ Have you had similar experience previously? Any other medical illness or surgeries?

◆ Do you smoke? Do you drink or use drugs?

◆ What about your blood sugar and blood pressure?

◆ Can I ask you some thing personal? Can you tell me about your sexual preferences?

◆ Where do you work?

◆ Anyone in your family with similar problems, any one with cancer of water bag or cancer of gland at the neck of water bag?

◆ Are you on any medication? Are you allergic to anything?

Is there anything else that you would like to tell me?

I appreciate your co-operation. Thanks and take care.

14. BLEEDING PER RECTUM

Mrs. Robert is 30 years old. She has come with complaints of bleeding from back passage. Elicit history from her.

Hello Mrs. Robert, how are you feeling? I am Dr. XYZ, Senior House Officer in Medicine. I am here to ask you few questions regarding your complaint so that we can find out what is causing it. Is that Ok with you?

◆ When did you first notice this problem?

Was it sudden or building up gradually?

Is it present every time you open your bowel?

Is it mixed with the waste or comes separately? How does it appear?

As a spot/as a streak/pours down/falls as a splash?

◆ Do you have itching in that region? **(Haemorroid)**

◆ Have you lost your weight? What about your appetite? Have you noticed any glands in your body? **(Cancer colon)**

◆ Do you feel that something pops out from your back passage whenever you strain? **(Rectal prolapse)**

◆ Do you have pain in the back passage? **(Anal fissure)**

◆ What about your bowel habits? Do you have any rashes on your body or joint pain? **(IBD)**

◆ Did you travel to any foreign places recently? **(Amoebic dysentery)**

◆ Have you had similar such experience in the past? Any other medical or surgical illness?

◆ Do you smoke? Do you drink or use drugs?

◆ What about your blood sugar and blood pressure?

◆ Can I ask you something personal? Are you in a stable relation? What about your sexual preferences?

◆ Where do you work?

◆ Anyone in your family with similar problems, any one with cancer of bowel or cancer of back passage?

◆ Are you on any medication? Are you allergic to anything?

Is there anything else that you would like to tell me?

I appreciate your co-operation. Thanks. I'll come back to you later.

15. HAEMATURIA

Here is a 65 years old male Mr. Samuel, who has come with passing blood in the water. Elicit detailed history from him.

Hello Mr. Samuel, how are you feeling? I am Dr. XYZ, Senior House Officer in Surgery. I am here to ask you a few questions regarding your complaint so that we can find out what is causing it. *Is that Ok with you?*

◆ When did you first notice this problem?

Did it start all of a sudden or has it been occuring since few days?

Does anything seem to worsen it? What makes you feel better?

Do you notice it every time when you pee? *urinate*

Is it initially when you pee or in the end or mixed with the water?

◆ Have you lost weight? What about your appetite?

Did you notice any glands in your body? **(Cancer bladder, cancer prostate)**

◆ Do you have running temperature? Do you have burning waterworks?

Do you have pain in the tummy? **(UTI)**

◆ Did you sustain any injury to the water pipe? **(Trauma)**

◆ Did you notice stones in your water?

Do you have problems with your water works? **(Stone)**

◆ Do you have difficulty in peeing? **(Prostate cause – BPH)**

◆ Did you notice any discharge from the water pipe? Any pain?

What about your sexual preferences? **(Gonorrhoea).**

◆ Did you travel to any foreign place? Any holidays recently and swimming? **(Schistosomiasis)** *— africa, Middle East, Indian Ocean.*

◆ Have you had similar experience previously? Any other medical illness or surgeries?

◆ Do you smoke? Do you drink or use any recreational drugs?

◆ What about your blood sugar and blood pressure?

- Anyone in your family with similar problems, any one with cancer of water bag?
- Where do you work?
- Are you on any medication? Are you allergic to anything?
  Is there anything else that you would like to tell me?
  I appreciate your co-operation. Thanks and take care.

OBSTETRICS AND GYNAECOLOGY

16. AMENORRHOEA

Mrs. Jenny has come to the gynaecology OPD with 9 months of amenorrhoea. Take history from her. She is 35 years old.

Hello Mrs. Jenny, how are you feeling? I am Dr. XYZ, Senior House Officer in Gynaecology. I am here to ask you a few questions regarding your complaint so that we can find out what is causing it. is it ok with you?

- When did you first have your periods? Have they been regular?
  When was your last periods? Could you be pregnant?
  Are you on pills or coil now?
- Are you experiencing any new changes within you, hot flushes, mood changes, dry sex? **(Menopause)**
- Are you worried about your weight? What type of clothes do you prefer? How many hours do you spend on exercise? **(Anorexia nervosa)**
- Are you stressed up a lot? Are you worried about your home, work, and family? **(Anxiety)**
- Are you running temperature? Do you have any discharge from the front passage? **(PID)**
- Have you noticed any change in your weight, any bloating sensation, increased hair growth on your face? **(PCOD)**
- Do you get headaches frequently? Any problems with vision? Do you have leaky breasts? **(Prolactinoma, brain tumour)**
- Did you visit any Asian country or come in contact with anyone with TB? **(Tuberculosis)**
- Did you undergo any X-ray therapy or any surgery of womb or egg producing gland?
  Anyone in your family attained menopause early? **(Premature menopause)**

- have any children, or was pregnant b4? (Asherman's / Sheehan's Syndrome)

◆ Is this the first time or have you had it previously also? Any other medical illness?

◆ Do you smoke? Do you drink or use drugs?

◆ What about your blood sugar and blood pressure?

◆ Can you tell me about your sexual preferences? Where do you work?

◆ Anyone in your family with similar problems?

◆ Are you on any medication? Are you allergic to anything?

Is there anything else that you would like to tell me?

I appreciate your co-operation. Thanks and take care.

NOTE:

1. If primary amenorrhoea rule out:

Physiological	PCOD
Imperforate hymen	Prolactinoma
Pregnancy	Anorexia nervosa
Pills	Tuberculosis
	Anxiety

17. BLEEDING PER VAGINUM

Mrs. Aldware is 38 years old and is complaining of excess bleeding per vaginum. Elicit history from her.

Hello Mrs. Aldware, how are you feeling? I am Dr. XYZ, Senior House Officer in Gynaecology. I am here to ask you a few questions regarding your complaint so that we can find out what is causing it. Is it ok with you?

◆ When did this start? Is it related to your periods? - endometriosis

Have your periods been regular?

When was your last period?

Are you on pills or coil? - ectopic

Could you be pregnant?

Do you have pain in the lower tummy? Was it the pain or bleeding which was first? Do you feel dizzy and sick?

Did you pass clots? **(Ectopic pregnancy/Abortion)**

◆ Do you have painful waterworks?

Do you have pain in the tummy?

Did you notice any mass? What about your waterworks? **(Fibroid)**

◆ Do you have pain during intercourse? **(Endometriosis)** PID (chlamydia coz deep dyspareunia)

◆ Do you have running temperature, pain or discharge down below? **(PID)**

◆ Is this bleeding related to intercourse? **(Cervical cause)** *cervical cancer, ectopion.*

◆ Do you feel you have lost your weight? What about your appetite? **(Cancer cervix)**

◆ Did you sustain trauma to the region of front passage? **(Trauma)**

◆ Have you had similar experience previously? Any other medical illness or surgeries?

◆ Do you smoke? Do you drink or use drugs?

◆ What about your blood sugar and blood pressure?

◆ Anyone in your family with similar problems, any one with cancer of breast, egg producing gland, womb, and neck of womb?

◆ Are you on any medication? Are you allergic to anything?

Is there anything else that you would like to tell me?

I appreciate your co-operation. Thanks and take care.

PAEDIATRICS

18. CHILD WITH FEVER

Mrs. Afflick has come to the A+E with her little one running high temperature and is worried. Take a detailed history from her.

Hello Mrs. Afflick. How are you? I am Dr. XYZ, Senior House Officer in Accident and Emergency. What has happened to the little one? *I will ask you few questions about your child so as to find out the cause. Is that ok with you?*

◆ Since when is she having running temperature?

Did you note the temperature?

Is it present continuously or intermittently?

◆ Has she been sick? Is she resenting light?

Does she have neck stiffness?

Is she feeding well? Is she breathing well?

Did you notice any rashes on her body?

When did it start? Has it increased in size?

Does it spread? Did you do the tumbler test? What happened after it? **(Meningitis)**

◆ What about her weight? Does she pee often? **(Diabetes mellitus)**

◆ Does she have pain in the tummy?

Does she have pain during passing water? **(UTI)**

◆ Does she have ear pain? Any discharge from her ears or nose? Does she have cold or cough? **(Otitis media, sinusitis)**

◆ Does she have runs? **(GIT upset)**

◆ Does she have fits? **(Febrile convulsions)**

◆ Has she taken all her jabs regularly?

◆ Is she a healthy child normally?

◆ Does she have any other medical illness?

◆ Is she on any medications or allergic to anything?

◆ Anyone else in the family with similar complaints?

Is there anything else that you would like to tell me?

We will take care of everything. Don't worry. Thanks for your co-operation. *I will be back to you later.*

19. INCESSANTLY CRYING CHILD

Mrs. Helen has got her 6 weeks baby boy being crying incessantly. The child is not at all consolable. Elicit relevant history from her and speak about the condition to her.

Hello Mrs. Helen. How are you? I am Dr. XYZ, Senior House Officer in Accident and Emergency. What has happened to the little one?

◆ When did it happen first?

How long does the episode last?

How many times has he had this?

Does anything worsen his condition?

What makes him feel better?

Does he cry continuously or intermittently?

◆ Does he lift his leg up during these episodes? *(>3hr, ≥ 3d/w – Cow's milk protein allergy).*
(Intussusception).

Does he become pale?

Has he been having problems opening his bowel?

Did you notice any lump in his tummy?

Did he pass blood with his waste? **(Intussusception)**

◆ Does he have running temperature?

Does he pee frequently?

Does he have any problem with waterworks? **(UTI)**

◆ Does he feel better when fitted with a seat belt in a car or when sitting on you? **(GERD)**

◆ Does he cry holding his ear? Did you notice any discharge from his ear? **(Ear pain)**

PLAB-2

- Has he received all his jabs regularly?
- Is he a healthy child normally? Any medical illness or surgeries?
  Is there anything else that you would like to tell me?
  We will take care of everything. Don't worry. Thanks for your co-operation.

NOTE:

More often the diagnosis is intussusception. The conversation should conclude by explaining the diagnosis and its management to the patient's mother/father.

"Mrs. Helen, little ABC has a condition called intussusception wherein the bowel telescopes into itself. First, we have to confirm this, which we will do by using a special X-ray. We will give fluids through his vein and carry on. Most of the time, the condition gets treated by non-surgical method, if not a paediatric surgeon will perform a surgery to correct it. We will do everything in the best interest of the little one. Thank you.

20. FEBRILE CONVULSIONS

Mrs. Xena has come with the little one running temperature and having fits. Elicit history and counsel regarding it.

Hello Mrs. Xena. How are you? I am Dr. XYZ, Senior House Officer in Accident and Emergency. What is the little one's name? I am here to ask you a few questions regarding the little one is that OK?

- Can you tell me if it was the temperature or fits first?
- When did she have running temperature?
  Did you check the temperature? What was it?
  Was it continuous or intermittent?
  Did you give any medications?
- After how many hours did she have fits?
  Did her whole body shake? Did she pee or open her bowel?
  Did she bite her tongue? Did she feel drowsy later?
- Did she have difficulty in moving her neck? Is she avoiding light?
  Did you notice any rashes on her body?   **(Meningitis)**
- How about sickness and her bowel habits?   **(GIT upset)**
- Has she got a cold or cough?   **(Respiratory tract infection)**
- Has she taken all her jabs to date?

◆ Is she a healthy child normally?

◆ Did she have any other medical illness? What about her growth and feeding habits?

◆ Is she on any medications or allergic to anything?

◆ Anyone else in the family with similar complaints? Anyone with epilepsy?

Is there anything else that you would like to tell me?

Well Mrs. Xena this is a condition called febrile convulsion. It is not a life-threatening one however. It is seen in children aged 6 months to 3 years. The exact cause is unknown.

It is very important to prevent the attack by controlling the temperature.

◆ You can give Paracetamol syrup 1 tsp full once in every 4 hours.

◆ Remove all warm clothing's, can leave the windows opened, and switch on the fan.

◆ Can also do tepid water sponging.

In case she has an attack:

◆ Get her away from danger first.

◆ Do not panic.

◆ Don't try to control fits.

◆ Once fits stops get her to the A+E or to the GP.

◆ We'll also teach you how to give the medicine through her back passage.

Is there anything else you would like to ask? Don't worry we'll take care of her. Thanks for your co-operation.

21. DIABETIC CHILD

Mrs. Jenny has come with her child who has been passing more water than usual. Take history and come to a relevant diagnosis.

Hello Mrs. Jenny. I am Dr. XYZ, Senior House Officer in Paediatrics. How are you? How is the little one? How old is she? I would like to ask you a few questions regarding the complaint so as to find out what is causing this. Is that OK?

◆ Since when is she having this problem?

Is that she pees frequently or she pees more than usual?

Does she wake up in the night to pee?

Does she drink more water? Does she wet the bed?

◆ Do you have any concerns about her weight and appetite?
   Does she complain of any itching sensation in her front passage or any discharge?
   Does anyone in your family have diabetes mellitus? **(Diabetes mellitus)**

◆ Does she have burning waterworks?
   Any running temperature?
   Does she have pain in the tummy? **(UTI)**

◆ Does she get headache very often? Does she feel sick and has reduced vision?
   Does she feel drowsy? **(Diabetes insipidus, ICSOL)**

◆ Did she sustain any head injury? **(Head injury)**

◆ Has she taken all her jabs regularly?

◆ Is she a healthy child normally?

◆ Did she have any other medical illness?

◆ Is she on any medications or allergic to anything?
   Is there anything else that?
   You would like to tell me? I will come back to you again.
   We need to run a few tests on her before coming to a diagnosis. Anyway, don't worry; we will take care of her. Thanks for your co-operation.

22. UTI

Hello Mrs. Jacobie. How are you? I am Dr. XYZ, Senior House Officer in Paediatrics. What's happened to the little one?

◆ Since when is the little one having this problem?
   Did it start all of a sudden?
   Does he cry when he pees? Does he have to strain a lot?
   Did he pass blood mixed with his pee?
   Does he have fever, tummy pain?
   Did he sustain any injury to his water pipe?
   Did he leak water any time?
   Has he had similar problems previously?
   Did you note the temperature?
   Any other medical or surgical illness?
   Is there anything else that you would like to tell me?

Well Mrs. Jacobie, we need to run a few tests on him to find out if it could be due to infection of waterworks. We will also give him medication accordingly. Meanwhile, he should have more of water, pee regularly and empty his water bag regularly. Don't worry; we will take care of him. Thanks for your co-operation.

23. DIARRHOEA

Mrs. Jaqlin has come to the Department of Paediatrics with the little one who is 5 months old and having few episodes of runs. Take history from her.

Hello Mrs. Jaqlin. I am Dr. XYZ, Senior House Officer in Paediatrics. How are you? How is the little one? How old is she? I would like to ask you a few questions regarding the complaint so as to find out what is causing this. Is that OK?

◆ Since when is she having runs?

    Is she breathing normally? Is she responding well?

    Is she drowsy or active?   — dehydration.

    Can you tell me how many times she has had runs?

    What is the color? Does it smell bad?

    Did it contain blood in it?

    Has she been sick?

◆ Has she got running temperature or pain in her tummy?

◆ Is she avoiding light? Does she have fits?

◆ Did you travel out recently?

◆ Do you feel that her lips are dry, she cries without tears and her tongue is also   — dehydration. dry?

◆ What about her feeding?

◆ Has she had similar experiences in the past?

◆ Is she a healthy child normally?

◆ Has she taken all her jabs upto date?

◆ Anyone in the family with similar problems?

◆ Did she have any other medical illness?

◆ Is she on any medications or allergic to anything?

    Is there anything else that you would like to tell me?

Well Mrs. Jaqlin, continue breastfeeding her and you can also give her DIORALYTE, the instructions been mentioned clearly over the pack.

I will come back to you again. Don't worry; we will take care of her. Thanks for your co-operation.

PSYCHIATRY

24. DEPRESSION

Mrs. Kate came for consultation after the death of her husband. She has always been feeling low. Elicit a history from her and come to a diagnosis.

Hello Mrs. Kate. I am Dr. XYZ, Senior House Officer in Psychiatry. I know that you are going through very bad time and the death of your husband might be a devastating blow. I would like to have a small talk with you. I am sure you will feel better after this.

◆ S - Did you have a good night **sleep** yesterday?
  What time did you wake up?
◆ A - What did you have for breakfast today?
  Are you having your meals/food regularly? **(Appetite)**
◆ W - Do you have any concerns about your **weight**? Have you lost your weight recently?
◆ E - Are you having the **energy** to do things as you used to do before?
◆ M - Do you feel very low often? **(Mood)**
◆ A - Are you able to carry on with your normal **activities** like social meetings, jobs etc.,
◆ I - Do you feel you have lost **interest** in your life?
◆ L - What do you feel the future has in store for you? **(Future life)**
◆ Have you had any thoughts of harming yourself or others? Do you feel you are controlled by someone?
◆ Is this the first time you are feeling low or have you had the similar feeling previously?
◆ Any other medical or psychiatric illness?
◆ Do you smoke, drink or use drugs?
◆ What about your blood pressure and blood sugar?
◆ Does anyone else in your family have similar problems?
◆ Are you on any medication? Are you allergic to anything?
  Is there anything else that you would like to tell me? I appreciate your co-operation.

Well Mrs. Kate, since you are going through depression, you will be needing treatment in the form of counselling and medication and we will be glad to help you. We are here only to help you. I appreciate your patience, I will come back again.

25. POST-NATAL DEPRESSION

Mrs. Debra is 23 years old and has come with low mood. It is 4 months since she delivered. She is worried. Elicit a history from her and come to a diagnosis.

Hello Mrs. Debra. I am Dr. XYZ, Senior House Officer in Psychiatry. How are you feeling? You seem to be feeling very low. How is your baby doing? Can we have a small talk, this will make you feel better I am sure. Also, whatever we speak will be confidential.

◆ How are you feeling since the birth of your baby? Are you feeling any better than before?

Do you prefer being lonely? Do you cry when alone?

Have you fed your baby?

Do you have any thoughts of harming yourself or your baby?

◆ Did you have a good night sleep yesterday? What time did you wake up? **(Sleep)**

◆ What did you have for breakfast today? Are you having your meals/food regularly? **(Appetite)**

◆ Do you have any concerns about your weight? Have you lost your weight recently? **(Weight)**

◆ Are you having the energy to do things as you used to do before? **(Energy)**

◆ Do you feel very low often? **(Mood)**

◆ Are you able to carry on with your normal activities like social meetings, jobs etc.? **(Activities)**

◆ Do you feel you have lost interest in your life? **(Interest)**

◆ What do you feel the future has in store for you? **(Future life)**

◆ Are you anxious about your baby's health?

◆ Is this your first baby? Are you happy about the little one?

Are you worried about your family or job?

Did you have any problems during the antenatal period?

Was it a normal delivery? Did you have to undergo more pain?

Do you have soreness in the front passage or pain?

◆ Do you feel someone else is controlling you?
◆ Have you felt similar way previously? Any other medical, psychiatric or surgical illness?
◆ Does anyone else in your family have similar features?
◆ Can I ask you something personal?
   Was this baby a planned one? Are your relations with your partner and family good?
   Are they getting along well with your baby? What about your sexual drive?
◆ Do you smoke, drink or use drugs?
◆ What about your blood pressure and blood sugar?
◆ Are you on any medication? Are you allergic to anything?
   Is there anything else that you would like to tell me? I appreciate your co-operation.

Well Mrs. Debra, what you are going through is postnatal depression, which is seen in few women after delivery. It is not life-threatening or dangerous. All you need is a break. Enjoy life, have fun. Go out with your partner; don't worry about your baby. He is doing well. Have nutritious food and plenty of juices. It is not a disease. So, don't worry. It will come back to normal in time. Just take care of yourself. We can offer you treatment in the form of counselling and medications.

26. PTSD

Mr. Penny had been to college with his friend on his, motor bike and met with an accident. His friend expired and now he is blaming himself for his friend's death. He is feeling very low. Elicit relevant history and counsel him.

Hello Mr. Penny. I am Dr. XYZ, Senior House Officer in Psychiatry. How are you feeling today? I know that you are going through bad time now. But, by sharing your feelings with someone, will surely make you feel better and we are here to help you. Can we talk about it?
◆ What actually happened?
   When did it occur?
◆ Are you feeling **guilty** for what has happened?
◆ Do you get **flashbacks** of the incident?
◆ Do you feel **at the edge** always?

◆ Did you have a good night sleep yesterday?
  What time did you wake up?

◆ What did you have for breakfast today?
  Are you having your meals/food regularly?

◆ Do you have any concerns about your weight? Have you lost your weight recently?

◆ Are you having the energy to do things as you used to do before?

◆ Do you feel very low often?

◆ Are you able to carry on with your normal activities like social meetings, jobs etc?

◆ Do you feel you have lost interest in your life?

◆ What do you feel the future has in store for you?

◆ Do you feel as if someone is talking to you, or controlling your thoughts and acts?

◆ Any other medical or psychiatric illness?

◆ I hope you would not mind me going a little personal – what about your sexual drive?

◆ Do you smoke, drink or use drugs?

◆ What about your blood pressure and blood sugar?

◆ Are you on any medication? Are you allergic to anything?
  Is there anything else that you would like to tell me? I appreciate your co-operation.

First and foremost, I want to tell you that this incident was not because of your carelessness, it was an accident and there is no reason for you to feel guilty. Accidents occur in this world. You did not plan it, so don't feel guilty about it. Are you willing to take treatment? We can offer you treatment in the form of counselling and medications. You can feel free to contact us at any moment.

Thanks for listening so patiently.

27. ALCOHOL HISTORY

Elicit alcohol history from Mr. Harold who is about to undergo a major surgery and his MCV values have been found to be very high. Find if there is dependency.

Hello Mr. Harold. How are you feeling? I am Dr. XYZ, Senior House Officer in Surgery. As far as I know you have come here for toe nail removal surgery and we ran a few tests on you before the surgery and one of them has been found to be very high, i.e. MCV. I would like to ask you a few questions to find out what is causing this. Is that OK with you?

♦ Where are you working? How is your work going on of late?

What do you do during weekends?

What about your family? Are you getting on well with them?

Are you concerned about your weight and appetite?

Do you get any burning pain in your chest or tummy quite often?

Can you describe a typical day of yours? What do you do in your leisure?

How frequently do you drink? How much do you take?

♦ C - Have you anytime felt that you have to **cut down** your drinks?

♦ A - Are your family and friends **annoyed** with these habits of yours?

♦ G - Do you feel **guilty** of this habit?

♦ E - Do you drink as soon as you wake up? **(Eye opener)**

♦ Do you feel you are neglecting your family and work?

♦ Do you take more than previous to obtain the same effect?

♦ Do you feel anything if you don't take drinks?

♦ Excess pounding of heart, shaking of hand, excess sweating, runs, blurring vision, anxiety, irritation, dizziness or anything else.

♦ Any other medical or surgical illness?

♦ Do you smoke or use recreational drugs?

♦ What about your blood pressure and blood sugar?

♦ What about your sexual life? Is it satisfactory?

♦ Are you on any medication? Are you allergic to anything?

Is there anything else that you would like to tell me? I appreciate your co-operation.

I will come back to you later. Take care. Bye.

28. CHILD ABUSE

Mrs. Penny has come here to the A+E with her 6 weeks baby girl with fracture femur and bruises all over his body. She is very much worried. Elicit a history from her and find out what is the cause.

Hello Mrs. Penny. How are you? I am Dr. XYZ, Senior House Officer in Accident and Emergency. I know that you are very much worried about the little one. I would like to talk to you about this to find out what is causing this.

◆ What actually happened?

When did it happen?

What did you do immediately?

Has she had any such injuries previously?

Where were you when this happened?

Who looks after her usually? Does anyone like a nanny or a baby-sitter or child carer take care of her?

Was this a planned pregnancy? Was it a normal birth? How is her growth according to you?

Has she taken all her jabs upto date?

Does she feed well, sleep well?

◆ Are there any other children in your family?

Is there any sibling rivalry?

◆ I would like to ask you something personal. It will be confidential.

Is your partner the little one's father? Does he get along well with her?

Do you get along well with him?

◆ Do you smoke, drink or use drugs?

Is there anything else that you would like to tell me? I appreciate your co-operation. Thank you and Bye.

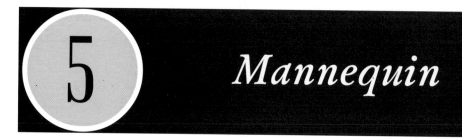

5 *Mannequin*

INTRODUCTION TO MANNEQUIN

Mannequins form an important part of the exams. Here address the mannequin indirectly through the examiner. Consider that you are doing the procedure on a live patient, taking care not to be rough. Here its our capacity to carry the procedure that will be examined.

The introduction in this case would be as follows.

"Ideally I would like to greet the patient, introduce myself, check the identity, build a rapport and explain the purpose of my visit. I will obtain consent, maintain utmost privacy and request the presence of chaperon." Then do the procedure and at the end thank all 3 (the patient, chaperon and the examiner).

1. CERVICAL SMEAR

There is a 26-year-old woman Jamie who has come with white discharge per vaginum. Obtain a cervical smear from her.

Good Morning, I'm Dr. ABC. (To the examiner)

Ideally, I would like to greet the patient, introduce myself build a rapport, check identity and mention the purpose of my visit. I'll request the presence of a chaperon. I'll explain the patient that I am here to take a sample of few cells from the neck of her womb and for this I need her to get undressed from below the waist behind the curtain and empty her water bag. I'll maintain utmost privacy and obtain a verbal consent. I will inform her I will be as gentle as possible.

Meanwhile, I'll check the trolley for a clean pair of gloves, Cusco's speculum, Ayre's spatula, slide, fixative, pencil, form, and warm water. I will write down the patient's name, inpatient number and date of birth on the slide.

I'll ask her to lie down on the couch on her back and to bend at her hip and knee and to keep her feet together and knee apart.

I'll ask her following:
1. If she is in her periods or having discharge from front passage.
2. If she could be pregnant.
3. If she had intercourse in the last 24 hours or used any lubricant.

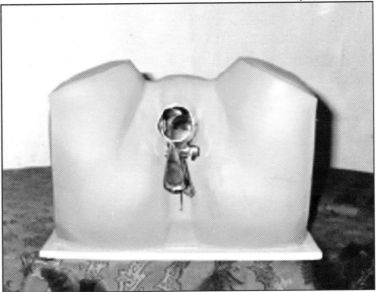

Figure 5.1: Per speculum examination

I'll explain her in detail and simultaneously wear my gloves, take the Cusco's and dip in warm water, check the warmth, separate the labia, inspect with light, introduce the speculum and fix it. I'll take the Ayre's spatula, introduce and at external os, rotate at 360°, remove it and spread it over the slide. Immediately use a fixative, keep slide in the box ready for dispatch, throw Ayre's into yellow bin and remove the speculum, (throw it if disposable into yellow bin or in tray if re-usable). I'll give her tissues and leave her in her privacy. I'll remove the gloves, put into yellow bin and fill the forms. I'll thank the patient for her co-operation and inform that we'll contact her as soon as the results are ready. I'll thank the chaperon. Thank you Doctor.

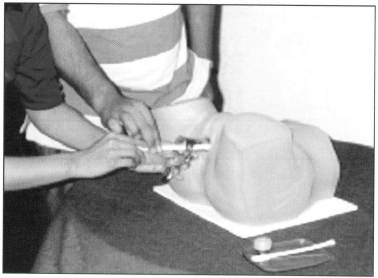

Figure 5.2: Cervical smear

NOTE:
1. Fill slide.
2. Ask questions.
3. Thank all the three.

2. PERVAGINAL EXAMINATION/BIMANUAL EXAMINATION

Mrs. Lorraine has come for a bimanual examination. Explain to her and do the procedure.

Good Morning, I'm Dr. ABC (To the examiner).

Ideally, I would like to greet the patient, build a rapport after introducing myself. I'll mention the purpose of my visit and also obtain a verbal consent. I'll request the presence of a chaperon. I'll explain that I'm going to introduce a finger into her front passage to examine and it may be of little discomfort. For this, she needs to get undressed from below the waist and also empty her water bag. I'll leave her in privacy to do this.

Meanwhile, I'll check the trolley if it contains a pair of clean gloves, swabs and lubricant. When she's back, I'll ask her to lie down on the couch on her back and bend at her hip and knee, to keep the feet together and knee apart.

◆ The distribution of pubic hair appears to be normal.

◆ Now, I'll inspect to see if there is any discharge or bleeding.

◆ There are no scars or sinuses or any redness that can be see.

◆ I'll place a kidney tray and ask her to cough, to see for prolapse or stress incontinence.

◆ I'll part the labia and see if there are any abnormalities in the clitoris. I'll see for the urethral opening.

◆ I'll feel for the bartholins gland at 5 and 7 o' clock position.

◆ I'll ask her to relax.

◆ Now, I'll insert 1 finger to feel the vaginal rugosity, if other finger can enter then I will insert second finger. I'm looking for any polyp or some growth in the vagina, if any.

◆ I can feel the cervix now, its firm in consistency. I can feel the external os, it's circular, and there are no growths that can be felt.

◆ Now, I'll feel for both right and left lateral fornix. Now, anterior fornix. There are no mass/growth attached or boggy mass. Now, posterior fornix for any fluid collection and tenderness.

◆ Now, I'm placing one of my hands over the tummy and feeling for uterus.

◆ Finally, I will do the cervical excitation test. I'll warn the patient that it may be painful and move the cervix to the right and left to elicit tenderness.

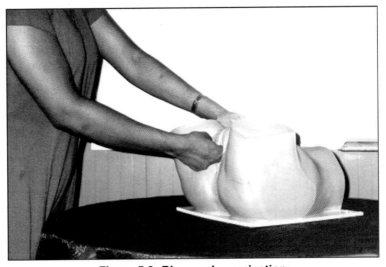

Figure 5.3: Bimanual examination

All the way through the examination, I'll keep a check on the patient to ensure that I'm not causing much discomfort.

I'll remove my finger now and give her wipes and leave her in privacy to get dressed.

I'll check for any discharge/blood on my finger and throw the gloves into the yellow bin.

I'll thank the patient. Thank the chaperon. Thank you doctor.

NOTE:
◆ Use the kidney tray without fail.
◆ If uterus felt, then its anteverted and if it is felt between the pubic symphysis and umbilicus, it is safer to tell that the size is 16–18 wks.

3. PERRECTAL EXAMINATION

Conduct per rectal examination explaining to the examiner what you are doing.

Good Morning. I'm Dr. ABC (To the examiner).

Ideally, I would like to greet the patient, introduce myself, check the identity, build a rapport and inform the purpose of my visit and the procedure. I'll request the presence of a chaperon. After obtaining consent from the patient, I'll ask him to undress from below the waist, to lie down on the couch on the left side with his knee and hip bent.

I'll explain that I will be introducing a finger into his back passage and I'll be as gentle as possible.

I'll check the trolley for clean pair of gloves, lubricant swabs and swipes.

I'll wear gloves, put gel on my index finger and ask him to breathe comfortably.
◆ I'll inspect the anus and ischiorectal region. I'll see if there are any excoriations, fissures, fistula and skin tag.
◆ I'll see for any sinus or discharge, bleeding from the anus.
◆ I'll put a generous amount of lubricant and place my index finger at the anal verge and move the index finger inside.
◆ I'll ask him to bear down and then squeeze my index finger to note the anal tone.
◆ Now, I'm seeing for the sacral curve, tenderness and any mass. Now, I'm feeling laterally.

◆ Now, I'm feeling for the rectal canal, for any mass, faecal matter.

Now, I'm turning my finger anteriorly.

1. I can feel the prostate.
2. Its firm is consistency.
3. The mucosa is slippery.
4. I can feel the lobes.
5. I can feel the median and lateral sulci.
6. The surface is smooth.
7. I can get above the prostate.

Now, I'll remove my finger and note if there is any discharge or blood and leave him in privacy to dress. I'll give tissues to wipe. I'll thank the patient for his co-operation. Thank the chaperon. Thank you.

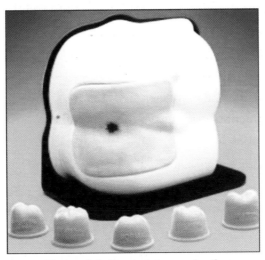

Figure 5.4: Perrectal examination

NOTE:

Character	Normal	BPH	Cancer
Consistency	Firm	Firm	Firm
Mucosa	Slippery	Slippery	Ir-regular
Lobes	Felt and regular	Shallow median sulcus/deep lateral sulcus	Cannot feel the sulcus, craggy surface.
Getting above	Can get above the prostate	Can't get above	Can/can't get above

4. OTOSCOPY

Good Morning, I'm Dr. ABC (To the examiner).

Ideally, I would like to greet the patient, introduce myself, check the identity, build a rapport and explain the purpose of my visit, i.e. to examine his ear. I'll proceed after obtaining consent.

◆ I'll explain that I would be examining his ear and during this procedure, my fingers will be touching his face. I'll introduce a torch-like instrument into his ear.

◆ I'll confirm that the instrument is working, i.e. the light and I'll use a new speculum.

◆ I'll see if there is any discharge from the ear, bleeding, sinus, scar, swelling, mastoid swelling.

◆ I'll feel for any swelling, then mastoid tenderness and tragal tenderness.

◆ I'll pull the pinna upward, backward and laterally.

◆ I can see the EAC, it's clear; there is no swelling, redness, foreign body, wax, and discharge. Now, I can see the tympanic membrane.
  1. It's pearly white–grey.
  2. I can see the cone of light.
  3. I can see the handle of malleus.
  4. There is no retraction/bulging.
  5. Can't see any fluid level.

To me, it appears to be normal tympanic membrane. I'll throw the aural speculum into yellow bin. Now, I would like to do Whispering test, Rinne's, Weber's. Due to time constraint, I'll do:

  • Modified Rinne's
  • Weber's

I'll take a high frequency tuning fork (512 Hz). I'll explain how the buzzing sound will be. I'll tell the patient, I'll place it in front of his ear and once behind his ear and will ask him to tell which sound he could hear better. I'll repeat it on the other ear also.

Now, I'll perform Weber's test, I'll explain that I'll keep the tuning fork on his forehead and he has to tell if he can hear equally in both the ears.

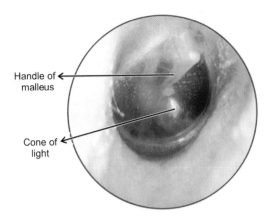

Handle of malleus

Cone of light

Figure 5.5A: Normal tympanic membrane

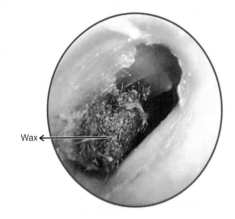

Wax

Figure 5.5B: Wax

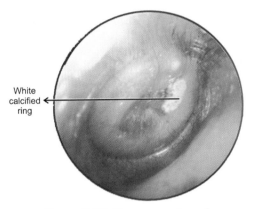

White calcified ring

Figure 5.5C: Tympanosclerosis

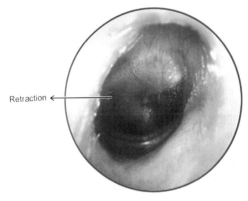

Retraction

Figure 5.5D: Middle ear infection (retraction)

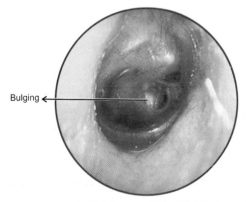

Bulging

Figure 5.5E: Middle ear infection (bulging)

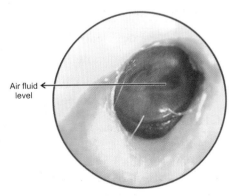

Air fluid level

Figure 5.5F: Middle ear effusion

PLAB-2

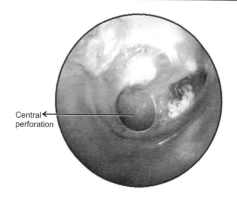
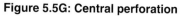

Figure 5.5G: Central perforation

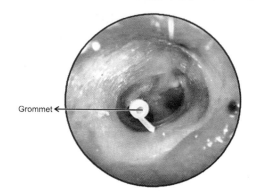

Figure 5.5H: Grommet

Then, I'll repeat the tests on the other ear. I'll request a senior to help me with the diagnosis.

I'll thank the patient for his co-operation.

Thank you Doctor.

NOTE:

1. **WAX**
   - ◆ I can't visualise the tympanic membrane.
   - ◆ The cone of light and handle of malleus are not visible.
   - ◆ My view is obscured by a foreign body, which is dark brown and glistening.
   - ◆ To me, it appears to be like wax.

2. **PERFORATION**
   - ◆ I can see the tympanic membrane (Grey white).
   - ◆ I can see the handle of malleus.
   - ◆ I can see a deficiency/hole in the tympanic membrane surrounded by normal tympanic membrane.
   - ◆ There is no discharge.
   - ◆ I think it is central perforation.

3. **GROMMET**
   - ◆ I can see the tympanic membrane, it's grey white.
   - ◆ I can see the handle of malleus.
   - ◆ I can see the cone of light as well.
   - ◆ There is a small white foreign body in the anterior inferior quadrant.
   - ◆ It appears to me like a grommet.

4. TYMPANOSCLEROSIS

◆ I can see the tympanic membrane, it's grey white.

◆ I can see the cone of light and handle of malleus.

◆ Around the tympanic membrane I can see a white ring.

◆ It appears to me as tympanosclerosis.

5. MIDDLE EAR INFECTION

◆ Congested tympanic membrane.

◆ Retracted/bulging.

◆ Level of fluid seen/not seen.

◆ Cone of light—Not visible.

6. MIDDLE EAR EFFUSION

◆ Tympanic membrane seen.

◆ Congested

◆ Handle of malleus and cone of light not visible

◆ Air-fluid level seen clearly.

5. OPHTHALMOSCOPY

Good Morning, I'm Dr. ABC (To the examiner).

Ideally, I would like to greet the patient, introduce myself, check the identity, explain the procedure and obtain consent. I'll maintain privacy and ask for a chaperon.

I'll inform that I will be examining the back of his eyes with a special torch-like instrument.

He has to look ahead without shaking his eyes. The lights will be switched off, i.e. the room will be made dark. A chaperon will be present during the procedure, I will be coming close to his face and my fingers may touch his forehead and cheek. The bright light from the torch may cause a bit of discomfort, but just for sometime.

◆ The distribution of eyebrow and eyelash is normal. There is no discharge, swelling or redness that is evident.

◆ I'll test if the light is working in the instrument.

◆ I'll stand at an arm's distance from the patient and holding the instrument with my right hand and viewing his right eye with my right eye.

   1. I can see the red reflex. Now, I'm going closer to the patient.

2. I'm seeing the optic disc
   - ◆ It's pale yellow.
   - ◆ It's round.
   - ◆ The margins can be made out clearly.
   - ◆ Cup-disc ratio appears to be normal.
   - ◆ I can trace blood vessels in the optic disc.
3. I can trace blood vessels in all 4 quadrants and also towards the optic disc.
4. The macula appears to be normal.
5. There are no haemorrhages or exudates seen.

It appears to be normal fundus.

I'll request my senior to help me with the diagnosis.

I will examine the other eye in similar fashion.

I'll remind the patient not to drive and not to sign important documents for a few hours if I have used a mydriatic.

I'll thank the patient for being co-operative. I'll thank the chaperon. Thank you Doctor.

NOTE:

1. HYPERTENSIVE RETINOPATHY
- ◆ The arteries are narrowed.
- ◆ The veins are compressed.
- ◆ Few haemorrhages can be seen.

2. DIABETIC RETINOPATHY
- ◆ Dot and blot haemorrhages are seen.
- ◆ Cotton wool spots seen.
- ◆ Hard exudates are seen.

3. NEOVASCULARISATION
- ◆ Many new blood vessels are seen.

4. PAPILLOEDEMA
- ◆ OD is pale and swollen.
- ◆ Margins of OD cannot be made out.
- ◆ Fundus is congested.
- ◆ Blood vessels are tortuous.

5. PHOTOCOAGULATION
- ◆ Many round white-yellow spots are seen.

6. **CRVO**
- Optic disc is not seen.
- Fundus is congested.
- Splashed tomato appearance.
- Blood vessels are engorged, veins congested.

7. **OPTIC ATROPHY**
- Optic disc is pale.

8. **CHRONIC SIMPLE GLAUCOMA**
- Mild cupping is seen.
- Cup is wider.

9. **SENILE MACULAR DEGENERATION**
- Unusual pigmentation present around macula, i.e. Drusen sign positive.

6. MEASURE BLOOD PRESSURE

Here is a 70-year-old man who has come with dizziness. History taken and now examine his blood pressure.

Hello, I'm Dr. ABC, Senior House Officer in Medicine. How are you today Mr. Wendall? I'm here to check your blood pressure and for this, I want you to roll your sleeve up and just relax.

Now, I'll tie this cuff, I want you to keep your arm straight. Did you have coffee or tea in the last ½ hour? Do you feel dizzy when you stand up suddenly? Do you have pain in the shoulder or elbow? Are you on any medication?

I will inflate the cuff with air and you will feel it as a tight constriction. I'll be as gentle as possible. Now, I'm checking radial pulse. I'm doing the palpatory method. Now, I'll do auscultatory method.

Can you please stand. Now, I'll check the blood pressure both methods again. I'll remove the cuff.

Thanks for your co-operation.

Thank you Doctor.

NOTE: Write the readings on a paper.

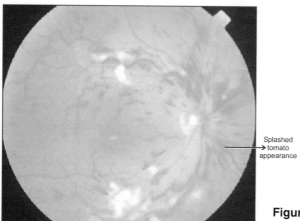

Splashed
tomato
appearance

Figure 5.6: CRVO

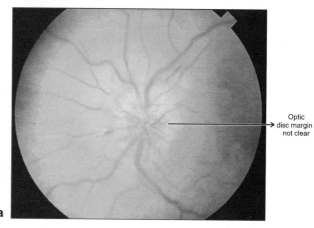

Optic
disc margin
not clear

Figure 5.7: Papilloedema

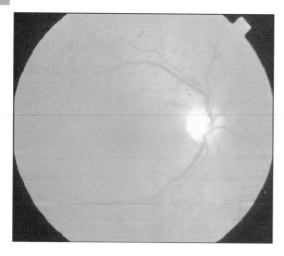

Figure 5.8: Diabetic retinopathy

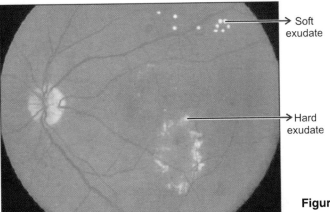

Soft
exudate

Hard
exudate

Figure 5.9: Diabetic retinopathy

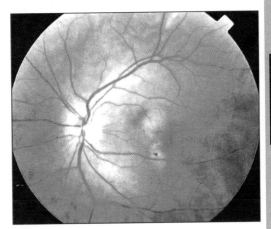

PLAB-2

Figure 5.10: Neovascularisation

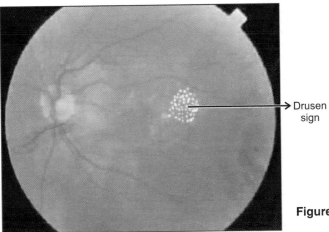

Drusen
sign

**Figure 5.11: Senile macular
degeneration**

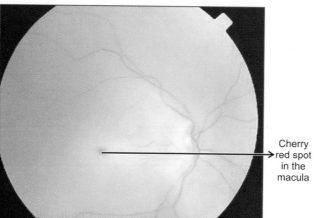

Cherry
red spot
in the
macula

Figure 5.12: CRAO

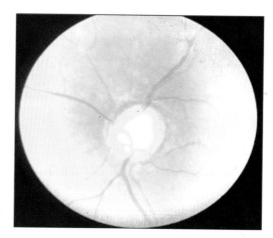

Figure 5.13: Optic atrophy

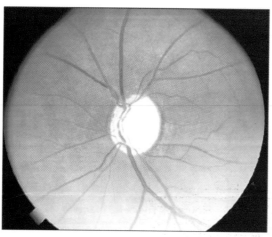

Figure 5.14: Glaucoma

7. BREAST EXAMINATION

Here is Mrs. Christopher who has come with pain in the right breast. Consent has been taken proceed.

Good Morning Mrs. Christopher. I'm Dr. ABC Senior House Officer in Surgery.

I'm here to examine your breast. I'll be as gentle as possible. You can tell me if I'm causing any discomfort. I will request for a chaperon and I'll ensure utmost privacy. For this, I need you to get undressed from neck to the waist.

On Inspection:
◆ Both breasts appear to be in the same level.
◆ The nipples are also at the same level, no discharge seen.
◆ The areola appears to be normal.
◆ Skin over has no ulcer, fissure, sinus, redness, and lesion.
◆ No obvious lump is seen.

Can you please place your hands over the hip and press tightly?
◆ No puckering seen.

Can you please raise your hand over your head?
◆ No puckering seen, no fullness in axillary fossa.

Can you please lift your breasts up?
◆ No lesions seen in the inframammary region.

Can you please bend forward?
◆ Both the breasts fall forward equally.

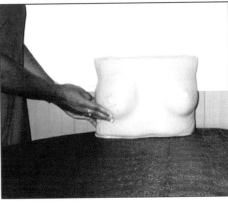

Figure 5.15: Breast examination

ON PALPATION

◆ Now I'll be touching you. I'm feeling for temperature and tenderness. I'm feeling in all 4 quadrants, areola, nipple, axillary tail. I'm feeling for any lump.

LYMPH NODES

◆ Anterior, posterior, medial, lateral, central (Axillary group of lymph nodes).

Ideally, I would like to examine the liver and spleen, the spine.

Thank you for your co-operation. You can get dressed now. I'll thank the chaperon.

Thank you doctor.

8. IV CANNULATION/VACUTAINER/BLOOD SAMPLING

Here is Miss Rudrocks who has come for blood sampling. She is suspected of being anaemic. Do the blood sampling. Do IV cannulation.

Ideally, I would like to greet the patient, introduce myself, check the identity, build a rapport, explain the purpose of my visit and also obtain a written consent. I'll explain that I'm here to put a small, thin tube into her vein and it will be like a scratch, but not painful. If I am not able to do it at first shot, then I may have to repeat it again. I'm not scaring you. I'll request the presence of chaperon.

◆ I'll check the site, where I will insert the cannula.

◆ I'll tie a tourniquet.

◆ Recheck the vein.

◆ Wear my glove. I'll use steret to swab the vein from distal to proximal.

◆ Use the cannula, remove it from the cover, and remove the cap.

◆ I'll stretch the skin downwards and with bevelled edge upwards, introduce the needle into the vein and wait for blood to show and further push the cannula and withdraw the needle. I'll remove the needle and throw into sharps bin and cover the cannula with cap. Apply a tape over the site.

I'll thank the patient for her co-operation. I'll thank the chaperon.

Thank you Doctor.

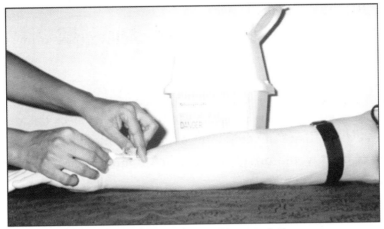

Figure 5.16: Intravenous cannulation

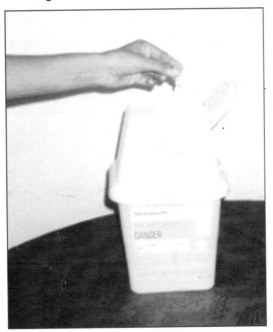

Figure 5.17: Sharps bin

NOTE:
- ANAEMIA   : FBC – EDTA
- DIABETES   : GLUCOSE – FLUORIDE
- JAUNDICE   : LFT – SST
- CHROMOSOMAL : LITHIUM HEPARIN
  STUDIES

PLAB-2

9. URINARY CATHETERISATION

Mr. Landoski is 70 years old and has come with inability to pass urine. Catheterise him and explain the procedure to the examiner.

Good Morning Doctor. I'm Dr. ABC (To the examiner)

Ideally, I would like to greet the patient, introduce myself, check the identity, build a rapport and explain that I'm here to put a thin tube into his water pipe to enable his waterworks. That would bring a lot of relief to him. For this I need him to get undressed from below the waist.

First, I would ask the presence of chaperon, obtain consent and ensure that it will be done under privacy.

I'll check the trolley for Foley's catheter, 10cc syringe, distilled water, syringe with lubricant jelly, antiseptic solution, swabs, swab holding forceps, sterile drape, urosac bag.

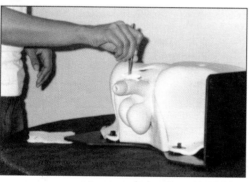 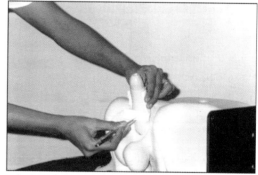

Figures 5.18A and B: Cleaning the area before catheterisation

- ◆ I'll ask him to relax.
- ◆ I'll clean the penis thoroughly, the suprapubic and medial aspect of the thigh. I'll warn the patient that it may be like stinging sensation when I install the medicine into his water pipe, but then it will facilitate to put the tube. Now, I'll hold the penis perpendicular to the couch and insert the lubricant jelly and ideally would like to hold for 5 minutes so that the jelly starts acting.
- ◆ Now, I'll take the catheter and insert it into the water pipe while holding the penis perpendicularly. Then, I will hold the penis at 45° and then insert until the Y junction. I'll place a tray down. I'll inject distilled water into the bulb and

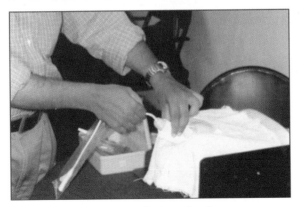

Figure 5.19: Catheterisation

fix it. Now I'll fix the catheter to the urosac bag.

◆ I'll tape the catheter to the medial aspect of thigh or the bed or the wheelchair.I'll ask him to get dressed.

I'll thank the patient for his co-operation and tell him not to worry, as we are there to take care of him.

10. SPACER DEVICE

Mrs. Thomas has come with her son for information regarding spacer device. Explain how to use it.

Hello Mrs. Thomas. I'm Dr. ABC, Senior House Officer in Paediatrics.

How are you feeling today? How is the little one? I'll be explaining you about this device. If you are not able to follow at any moment, you can stop me at any point.

This is a spacer device. It is made of plastic and has two conical parts. One end has a slot for inhaler. This part, which has a beak like opening is mouthpiece and this, is where the little one will keep his mouth. This is how you fix it. Can you do it once for me? That's great.

You have to make him sit on your lap with his back facing your chest and hold the device in front of him and ask him to place his lips around the mouthpiece and ask him to breathe normally. Now, shake the inhaler well, remove the cap and spray once in air, place it in the slot and press the inhaler. The medicine will move through the chamber and reach the valve and then, when he breathes in, the medicine enters his lungs. Allow him to take normal breath for a minute. You can use the inhaler as prescribed. You have to get a new device when the sound of the valve stops. Now, I would like to tell about the cleaning aspects.

◆ You have to allow tap water to run through the device, drip dry or sun dry– once in a week.

◆ Do not scrape or scratch it.

The advantages of this device are:

◆ There is no need to co-ordinate the breathing.

◆ You can also use a mask if needed.

◆ The chance of infection in the mouth and throat is less.

◆ The amount of medicine used is less and it goes directly into the lungs.

The only disadvantage is that it is clumsy to carry the device. So ensure that the school nurse has one.

Have I answered all your queries, is there anything else?

You can feel free to contact us at any time.

Take care. Thank you.

11. PEFR

Mr. Chivas has been admitted with acute severe asthma and is now ready to be discharged. The inhaler technique has been explained to him already. Its necessary to monitor the PEFR. Explain him in detail.

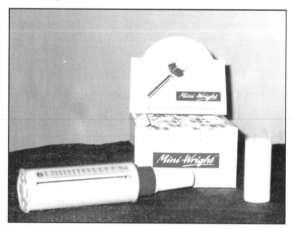

Figure 5.20: PEFR meter and disposable mouthpiece

Hello Mr. Chivas. I'm Dr. ABC, Senior House Officer in Medicine. How are you feeling? I'm glad you have recovered well and are going home.

I'm here to explain about this instrument called PEFR meter, which is important as we can get to know how well the medicine is acting on you and how well you are responding to it.

This is made of plastic and has a mouthpiece, which is disposable. This has readings here with a movable needle. You have to use it once in the morning and once in the evening. Every time you use it, make sure you use it three times, i.e. three blows. You have to stand straight, hold the meter horizontally and blow through the mouthpiece – AS FAST AS YOU CAN, AS MUCH AS YOU CAN AND AS HARD AS YOU CAN.

Make sure the needle is at 'O' every time you blow. Now, repeat the whole procedure another two times. Note the values, i.e. best of 3 and not the average. Discard the mouthpiece.

Do you have any doubts regarding this?

I would be glad to help you. Thanks for your co-operation. We'll meet again in the next appointment.

Take care and bye.

12. SUTURING

Miss Catherine had met with an accident today morning and she has a 4 cm cut over her arm. Put suture. You need to clean the wound and also anaesthetise the site. Consent has been obtained. Explain the procedure as you proceed.

Good Morning.

Ideally, I would like to greet the patient, introduce myself, check the identity and build a rapport. I'll explain to her that I'll clean the wound and give an injection that will make the area go numb and then I'll put a few stitches to enable quicker healing. I'll request a chaperon. I'll obtain written consent.

I'll check the trolley for anaesthetic solution, 10cc syringe (2); antiseptic solution, distilled water, suture material, swabs, needle holding forceps, toothed forceps.

PLAB-2

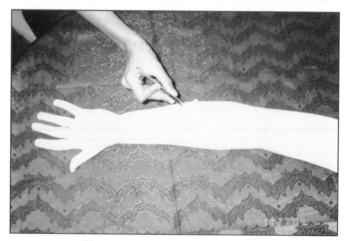

Figure 5.21: Cleaning the wound

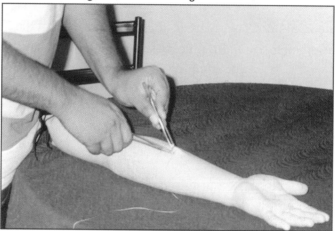

Figure 5.22: Suturing

I'll wear my gloves and first clean the wound with distilled water and then with antiseptic solution. I'll clean around the wound in circular fashion. Now, I'll remove the glove, wash hands and wear another pair. Take the local anaesthetic and warn the patient that she may feel stinging sensation for a few seconds. Ideally, I'll wait for 5 minutes. Now, I'll check if the anaesthetic is acting. Now, I'll request the nurse to open the suture pack and then put suture.

Repeat the same suture 5-10 mm apart.

I'll thank the patient for her co-operation. I'll advice her regarding suture removal and analgesics.

Thank you.

13. SAMPLE FOR ARTERIAL BLOOD GAS ANALYSIS

Collect blood from the patient Mr. Swelte for ABG analysis.

Good morning doctor.

Ideally I would like to greet the patient, introduce myself, check the identity, build a rapport and explain the purpose of my visit. I will obtain his consent and request the presence of a chaperon.

I will explain that I am here to collect a small amount of blood from him. I will be introducing a thin needle into his forearm and he may experience some pain but that will last for few minutes only.

I will check the trolley for a syringe, which is coated with heparin, the forms, steret, and clean pair of gloves.

I will wear the gloves and then feel for the pulse (radial artery or brachial artery or femoral artery).

Clean the site with the steret.

Now I will feel for the pulse again with my index and middle fingers.

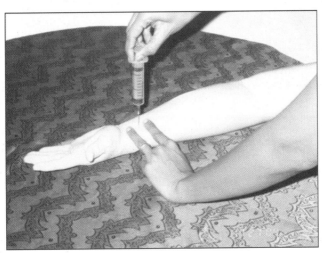

Figure 5.23: ABG analysis

At the junction of midpoint of these fingers towards the middle finger, where maximum or strong pulsation is felt is the point where I will be passing the needle perpendicularly.

Once inside the artery withdraw 1.5 ml of blood.

Remove the needle and then I will ask the patient or request the nurse to apply firm pressure over the site for sometime to prevent bleeding.

Cover the syringe with its cap and send it immediately to the lab for analysis. Taking care to send it on ice pack.

Apply pressure over the puncture site and a sterile gauze to prevent any bleeding from occurring further.

Thank the patient for his co-operation and tell him that we will contact him as soon as the results are ready.

Thank the chaperon and the examiner.

NOTE:

1. The syringe should be coated with heparin or any other anticoagulant in order to prevent clotting of the blood.
2. The analysis should be done immediately and infact it forms our duty to inform the laboratory even before the procedure.
3. Take care that there is no over dilution of the heparin and that there are no air bubbles in the sample as all these results in false readings.

PLAB-2

6 *Counselling*

INTRODUCTION TO COUNSELLING

This section tests our communication skills and how we can explain the medical details to the patient in layman terms. It is important that the patient understands everything in detail.

Obtaining Consent

Here you have to explain the procedure in detail the advantages and disadvantages, the need of the procedure, the preoperative intraoperative and postoperative details. Provide him with the leaflets and then consent form at the end.

Explain Diagnosis

Here explain all about the illness, what it is, what the features are, the problems that can arise, the tests for it, the treatment that is available and the course of the illness. Finally provide him with leaflets.

Medication Advice

About medication, explain the need of the medicine, the dosage, the mode of intake, duration, the action of the medicine and its side effects. Things to be cautious about while taking the medicine.

Breaking Bad News

This could be tough if not planned and prepared properly. Understand the situation well and then approach the station with sympathy. Keep your tone low. Never hide anything, break the news gently and tell the stage as well, whether its curable or incurable. Never give false hopes. Tell them everything straight forward give them the options that are available. Pause in between the discussion.

SECTION 1—OBTAINING CONSENT FOR PROCEDURES

1. ENDOSCOPY

Mr. Denny has come to surgery OPD with pain in the tummy which has not reduced after medication counsel regarding endoscopy.

Hello I am Dr. X, Senior House Officer in Surgery. How are you feeling today Mr. Denny? As you know, you have been troubled a lot due to this pain in the tummy since a long-time and had not been benefited with our medications, so we need to find out the cause, which we would like to do by a simple and common procedure that is Endoscopy. I am here to explain you everything in detail and also to answer all your questions about it. If you are not able to follow, you can stop me at any moment. Is that OK?

In this procedure we are going to introduce a thin tube that has a camera on its end, into your foodpipe.

You will have to fast 8 hours prior to the procedure and come to us .We will use a spray on to your throat or we will put you to sleep after giving you an injection. The procedure is going to last for few minutes.

We will introduce the tube into your mouth and then to your throat and foodpipe, later stomach. We will check if there is anything abnormal and then take a piece of the tissue if needed which is not going to be painful at all and then we will send it for further examination after removing the tube.

After this you can go home but you need someone to drive you back if we are using the injection and also you need someone to take care of you that night.

Are there any problems with this procedure?
Well this is a common problem and rarely causes any unwanted effects.
1. There may be mild discomfort, which will wear off by itself.
2. There may be small tears, which will heal off by itself rarely needing antibiotics or stitches.
3. Minimal bleeding.

What if I do not want to undergo this procedure?
This is going to help us to find out what actually the problem is and to plan our treatment further.

We are thinking only in the betterment of your health.

Is there anything else that you would like to know?

I would be glad to help you.

I will provide you with the necessary leaflets and information sheets that you can go through and if fully satisfied you can sign the consent form.

I appreciate your co-operation. Take care, Bye.

2. COLONOSCOPY

Mr. Davish was admitted with losing weight and problems with bowel. Counsel regarding colonoscopy.

Hello I am Dr. X, Senior House Officer in Surgery. How are you feeling today Mr. Davish?

As you know you have been troubled a lot due to this problem in your bowel and losing weight since a long-time and after running the tests we were not able to come to a diagnosis, so we need to find out the cause which we would like to do by a simple and common procedure that is colonoscopy. I am here to explain you everything in detail and also to answer all your questions about it. If you are not able to follow you can stop me at any moment. Is that OK?

In this procedure we are going to introduce a thin tube that has a camera on its end, into your back passage.

You will have to fast 8 hours prior to the procedure and we will give you few tablets to empty your bowel. We will make the area go numb or we can put you to sleep so that you will feel no discomfort at all. The procedure is going to last for few minutes. We will check if there is anything abnormal and then take a piece of the tissue if needed which is not going to be painful at all and then we will send it for further examination after removing the tube.

Are there any problems with this procedure?

Well this is a common problem and rarely causes any unwanted effects.

1. There may be mild discomfort that will wear off by itself.
2. There may be small tears which heals off by itself rarely needing antibiotics or stitches.
3. Minimal bleeding.

What if I do not want to undergo this procedure?

This is going to help us to find out what actually the problem is and to plan our treatment further.

We are thinking only in the betterment of your health.

Is there anything else that you would like to know?

I would be glad to help you.

I will provide you with the necessary leaflets and information sheets that you can go through and if fully satisfied you can sign the consent form.

I appreciate your co-operation. Take care, Bye.

3. FEMALE STERILIZATION

Counsel Mrs. Rennet who is 33 years old with 4 children regarding sterilization.

Hello I am Dr. X, Senior House Officer in Gynaecology. How are you feeling today Mrs. Rennet?

As far as I know you are here to know about the sterilization procedure and I am here to explain you everything in detail and also to answer all your questions about it. If you are not able to follow you can stop me at any moment. Is that OK? Before I can proceed would like to ask you a couple of questions.

◆ Are you sure you do not want any more children?

◆ Are you aware of the pills, coil and vasectomy?

◆ Could you be pregnant now?

Well, you will have to fast overnight and come to us on the day of surgery and you will be put to sleep regarding which, my anaesthetic colleague will speak to you in detail.

We will do the procedure as a keyhole operation or in the standard way where in a small nick will be made on the lower tummy and through this we will enter the tummy and identify the tubes and then put clips around each tube. This prevents the eggs from coming and meeting the sperms and hence prevents the pregnancy from occurring.

The procedure lasts for 30 minutes to an hour and you will be taken to the recovery room following this and once you are fine you will be discharged. There should be someone to take care of you that night.

This is a permanent procedure for all practical purposes and you should continue using the coil or pills until your next periods.

Are there any problems with this procedure?
I do not mean to scare you but I am duty-bound to explain this as well to you. There may be a few unwanted effects, which is not necessary that it should occur.
◆ There are chances of injury to the bowel, womb.
◆ Sickness and feeling sick due to anaesthesia, but it will wear off by itself.
◆ You may yet become pregnant and it would be an ectopic pregnancy.
◆ Rare chances of failure.
◆ Your periods may become painful and heavier.

What if I do not have children at all and want to undergo this procedure?
Its better to think well before this as the reversal rate is quite less.

Is there anything else that you would like to know?
I would be glad to help you.
I will provide you with the necessary leaflets and information sheets that you can go through and if fully satisfied you can sign the consent form.
I appreciate your cooperation. Take care, Bye.

4. VASECTOMY

Mr. Matt is very much interested in vasectomy. Counsel him regarding this procedure.

Hello I am Dr. X, Senior House Officer in Surgery. How are you feeling today Mr. Matt?
As far as I know you are here to know about vasectomy and I am here to explain you everything in detail and also to answer all your questions about it. If you are not able to follow you can stop me at any moment. Is that OK? Before I can proceed I would like to ask you a couple of questions.
◆ Are you sure you want to undergo this procedure?
◆ Have you spoken to your partner about this?

This is a permanent procedure for all practical purposes.

You will have to come here on the day of the procedure, you will not be put to sleep but the area where we are going to operate will be made to go numb.

We will make a small nick on the upper part of the scrotum on both the sides and then after identifying the vas, that is the sperm tube which carries the sperm to the outer world, will be cut, turned away from each other and then tied.

This will prevent the pregnancy. The operation lasts for 30-45 min and then stitches will be put over the skin and if everything goes fine you will be discharged home the same day.

You need someone to drive you back and to look after you when you are at home.

Do you have any queries to ask?

Will this operation cause any problem?
I hope I am not scaring you but I am duty-bound to explain you this in detail.
◆ You may experience some discomfort and this will wear off by itself, you can also use tight underpants to prevent this.
◆ There may be minimal pain for which we can give painkillers.
◆ Collection of blood beneath the skin, which will wear off by itself.
◆ Rare chances of failure.

Will this hinder with my sexual life?
No, not at all, it is not going to affect your manliness in anyway.
It is important that you follow some other mode of contraception for a period of at least 3 months until the smear reports of your semen prove to be negative.
You can resume with your activities after 1 week.
Your sex life will not be affected.

Is the surgery reversible?
It is reversible but the success rate is very low.

Is there anything else that you would like to know?
I would be glad to help you.
I'll provide you with the necessary leaflets and information sheets that you can go through and if fully satisfied you can sign the consent form.
I appreciate your cooperation. Take care, Bye.

5. HIP JOINT REPLACEMENT

Mr. Jones is 56-year-old and working as a teacher. Counsel him regarding hip joint replacement for the osteoarthrosis he has.

Hello I am Dr. X, Senior House Officer in Surgery. How are you feeling today Mr. Jones?

As far as I know you had problems with walking and lots of pain and I am here to explain you everything in detail and also to answer all your questions about it and to let you know what we are planning is the best for you? If you are not able to follow you can stop me at any moment. Is that OK?

Our consultant has decided to get the surgery done which is hip joint replacement.

Its very important for you to undergo this operation, as this will enable you to walk better and you can be as normal as you were previously.

How are you going to go about this surgery?
You will have to fast overnight and come to us on the day of surgery. You will be put to sleep and regarding this our anesthetist colleague will speak to you in detail. You will be taken to the operation room and a nick of 5-7 inches will be made on the upper and outer aspect of your thigh.
Through this we will remove the diseased joint and replace it with artificial joint. The operation lasts for 2 hours or so and stitches will be put and a rubber tube will be coming out from the operated site to remove if there is any discharge.
You will be taken to the recovery room and given painkillers into your blood through a thin tube along with fluids. And a tube will be passed into your water pipe to drain the water, which will remain for 2-3 days.
You can start off with movements after 2-4 days initially on frames and later on crutches and we'll monitor you. A physiotherapist will be referred to help you with your movements and exercises.

Is it really necessary to undergo this surgery?
Yes, its very much needed as we are thinking for the betterment of your health and you will be able to walk as before and without pain.

PLAB-2

I have heard that the operation may cause some problem, what do you think about it?

Well the unwanted effects are not seen in all the patients whom we operate and I am duty bound to explain that as well.

◆ You may experience sickness and it's due to the anesthesia and it will wear off by itself.

◆ Pain for which we will give painkillers.

◆ Infection for which there are antibiotics.

◆ There is a possibility of formation of clot in the leg, for this we can give blood thinners.

◆ Rare chances of loosening of prosthesis, that is, the artificial joint.

You will be seen by your GP regularly.

Stitches will be removed after 2 weeks time once the wound is fine.

The prosthesis will last for 10-12 years.

Is there anything else that you would like to know?

I would be glad to help you.

I'll provide you with the necessary leaflets and information sheets that you can go through and if fully satisfied you can sign the consent form.

I appreciate your cooperation. Take care, Bye.

6. COLOSTOMY

Mr. Zelweger has been admitted with intestinal obstruction talk to him about colostomy (only colostomy).

Hello I am Dr. X, Senior House Officer in Surgery. How are you feeling today Mr. Zelweger?

As far as I know you had problems with opening your bowel and I am here to explain you everything in detail and also to answer all your questions about it and to let you know what we are planning is the best for you? If you are not able to follow you can stop me at any moment. Is that OK?

After thorough examination and running a few tests our consultant has decided to do Colostomy. The obstruction in your bowel is not allowing the poo to pass out and this if left as it is can further result in infection that can spread through out the body which inturn can become life threatening. The best would be to undergo this surgery.

Here in you will have to fast overnight and come to us on the day of surgery and you will be put to sleep regarding which, our anesthetic colleague will speak to you in detail. We will make a nick of about 1-2 inches on the tummy in the left side and then through this we will approach the bowels and then get the bowel out in the form of a spout and put few stitches so that its fixed to the skin and its end would be connected to an opaque and disposable plastic bag. The procedure itself will last for around 1-2 hours.

After this you will be taken to the recovery room and given painkillers. If everything goes out fine you will be discharged after 3-5 days.

A special nurse called stoma nurse will take care of you and also will teach you about the care of the wound. You will have to attend the stoma clinic regularly. The bag that we connect to the spout is a thin one and will not be visible to a near by person.

Are there any problems associated with this surgery or after it?
Well, as in any surgery there may be a few complications, which usually are rare and also manageable.
◆ You may have sickness or you may feel sick, this being due to anesthesia and it will wear off by itself.
◆ Your bowel frequency may increase for the first few days after the surgery and this is only till your body gets used to this new change.
◆ In case there is any infection we will give you antibiotics.
◆ There may be mild excoriation at the wound site and even shrinkage of the wound.
◆ Minimal bleeding.
I can understand that this is very anxious moment for you, but we are thinking only in terms of your benefit.
You can resume with your normal activities once the wound heals, you can start with your driving after 2-3 weeks.
Your sex life will not be affected which you can resume once the wound site heals.

Is there anything else that you would like to know?

I'll provide you with the necessary leaflets and information sheets that you can go through and if fully satisfied you can sign the consent form.

I appreciate your cooperation. Take care, Bye.

7. TERMINATION OF PREGNANCY

Miss Catherine has come for termination of pregnancy after mild bleeding from front passage. Explain to her regarding it.

Hello I am Dr. X, Senior House Officer in Obstetrics. How are you feeling today Miss. Catherine?

As far as I know you had come to us to terminate your pregnancy and I am here to explain you everything in detail and also to answer all your questions about it and to let you know what we are planning. If you are not able to follow you can stop me at any moment. Is that OK?

Do you have the pain and bleeding even now? Are you comfortable?

Before we can actually proceed we need to rule out if you have any infection?

Do you get headaches frequently? Have you had any pain in your legs?

Are you at the moment on coil or pills?

There are 2 different approaches:

1. *Medical method* where in tablets or pessary will be given and this will cause cramp like pain in your tummy similar to that of the pain during periods, with bleeding from the front passage and thus terminating the pregnancy. If the termination is not complete then we need to carry on with surgical method.

2. *Surgical method* is one where in you will be put to sleep and taken to the operation theatre and then we will gently suck the pregnancy out with a syringe. There are rare chances of injury to the womb by this method and bleeding as well.

After this procedure once you are feeling fine you can go home but you need someone to drive you back and to take care of you that night.

We need to do few blood tests to know your Rh status. We can put you on contraception if you need.

Is there anything else that you would like to know?

I would be glad to help you.

I'll provide you with the necessary leaflets and information sheets that you can go through and if fully satisfied you can sign the consent form.

I appreciate your cooperation. Take care, Bye.

8. OVARIAN CYSTECTOMY

Mrs. Catherine is 32-year-old and was diagnosed as having a big cyst in the ovary. Counsel her regarding ovarian cystectomy.

Hello I am Dr. X, Senior House Officer in Obstetrics. How are you feeling today Mrs. Catherine?

As far as I know you had come to us with pain in the tummy and after examining you thoroughly and running a few tests we have diagnosed it as a cyst in the egg producing gland and I am here to explain you everything in detail and also to answer all your questions about it and to let you know what we are planning. If you are not able to follow you can stop me at any moment. Is that OK?

Are you comfortable?

What is a cyst?

A cyst is similar to a balloon filled with water and in your case it is in the egg-producing gland and if it were to be a small one then we could have left it as it is but in your case it is big and this needs to be removed.

If it is left as it is, then there are high chances that it may burst open or it may twist on itself or it may cause bleeding and all of these will result in life threatening complications. The surgery itself is hence necessary.

Can you tell me how you are going to carry about with the surgery?

Sure, you need to fast over night and come to us on the day of surgery and our anesthetic colleague will speak to you in detail regarding this and then we will perform the surgery as a keyhole procedure. Here in, we will make small holes on your tummy and through one we will introduce the telescope with a camera fixed to its end and then we will introduce a harmless gas into the tummy and this is to view the organs clearly. This gas will be removed at the end of the procedure. Through the other hole the instrument will be introduced and then the cyst will be removed out. We will also see to it that the ovaries are fine. In case we find that there is any abnormality then we may have to remove the egg-producing gland as well. We will also check the gland on the other side before putting the stitches.

The procedure lasts for around 60 minutes and then you will be taken to the recovery room after the procedure.

If all goes well you will be discharged in 3-5 days time.

You can resume with your normal work in about 3-4 weeks time and also with your driving by the same time.

Your sex life will not be affected at all.

Are there any unwanted effects due to this surgery?

Well, I hope I am not trying to scare you but then I'm duty bound to explain you this as well. The complications are rare and are treatable as well.

1. You may experience sickness and it's due to the anesthesia and it will wear off by itself.
2. Pain for which we will give painkillers.
3. Infection for which there are antibiotics.
4. Chances of injury to the bowel are rare.

You will be followed regularly by your GP.

Is there anything else that you would like to know?

I would be glad to help you.

I'll provide you with the necessary leaflets and information sheets that you can go through and if fully satisfied you can sign the consent form.

I appreciate your cooperation. Take care, Bye.

9. MASTECTOMY

Mrs. Richter was diagnosed as cancer right breast, its stage 1 cancer; counsel her regarding mastectomy.

Hello I am Dr. X, Senior House Officer in Surgery. How are you feeling today Mrs. Richter?

As far as I know you had come to us with a lump in your right breast and after examining you and running a few tests we have diagnosed it as cancer of the breast but it is in the early stage and can be treated by a surgery and I am here to explain you everything in detail and also to answer all your questions about it and to let you know what we are planning is the best for you? If you are not able to follow you can stop me at any moment. Is that OK?

Now if left then there are high chances of this cancer to spread further and to involve other parts of the body and the other breast as well and at that stage it would become difficult to treat you as well and this could also result in further complications.

How are you going to carry about with the surgery?

You will have to fast overnight and come to us on the day of surgery and you will be put to sleep, regarding this our anaesthetic colleague will speak to you in detail. Our consultant will operate and remove the entire right breast that is affected. We can do a reconstructive surgery by putting an implant beneath the chest muscle and giving you the normal shape of the breast and the nipple. This we can do at the same sitting or at a different sitting.

The procedure may last for about 1-1.5 hours and we will put the stitches and then take you to the recovery room. Here we will give you adequate painkillers and necessary fluids.

You'll have to stay here in the hospital for 3-5 days and then can go home. You need to take rest for at least 2-3 weeks. You can resume with driving from 3-4 weeks onwards. You will be followed regularly by your GP.

There is going to be no problem with your sex life.

Will there be any problems following this surgery?

Well the unwanted effects are not seen in all the patients whom we operate and I am duty bound to explain that as well.

1. You may experience sickness and it's due to the anesthesia and it will wear off by itself.
2. Pain for which we will give painkillers.
3. Infection for which there are antibiotics.
4. There is a possibility of formation of clot in the leg, for this we can give blood thinners.

Can you tell me something about the implants?

Sure, there are 2 types of implants:

External implants: Cotton or Woollen pads.

Padded brassieres.

Night wear and swim suits that are padded.

Internal implants: Muscle tissue taken from your body itself, which will be replaced in the place of the removed breast.
Silicon implants.

You will be followed regularly by your GP.
Is there anything else that you would like to know?
I would be glad to help you.
I'll provide you with the necessary leaflets and information sheets that you can go through and if fully satisfied you can sign the consent form.
I appreciate your cooperation. Take care, Bye.

SECTION 2—MEDICATION ADVICE

1. ANTIEPILEPTIC MEDICATION

Counsel regarding carbamazepine to Miss. Jane. She is 22-year-old university student.

Hello, I am Dr. X Senior House Officer in Psychiatry. How are you feeling today Miss. Jane? As far as I know you had come to us with fits and we had diagnosed it as Epilepsy and I am sure you are aware of it. Well now I am here to tell in detail about the medication that you need to take and everything about it. In case you are not able to follow you can stop me at any moment and I will be glad to explain you again. Is that OK?

Well, the condition occurs due to the abnormal electrical discharge from the brain.

We will give you this medicine Carbamazepine that you have to take regularly without stopping unless we tell you to. Take it as 1 tablet in the morning and 1 in the evening for the first 2 weeks and from third week onwards its 2 tablets in the morning and 2 tablets in the evening. Remember that you should take it at particular timings of the day. For example you can consider taking it exactly at 8.00 in the morning and 8.00 in the evening. Take care that you don't stop these medications or forget to take them because the fits may return if you do so.

We will have a regular check on your blood for the amount of medicine in your blood and then decide further if it is necessary to change the dosage.

driving: ① Seizure while awake, must not drive for 1yr.
② attacks while sleeping, stop driving for 1yr, unless attack was while sleepin & > 3yrs ago & there have not been any awake fits since that asleep attack.
③ cease driving from the beginning of withdrawal & not recommence until

Counselling   89

I now would like to mention about the unwanted effects that the medicine could have though it's not necessary but it's my duty to explain this as well. Finally it's the benefits that we should be bothered about.

◆ Sickness and feeling sick

◆ Dizziness

◆ Double vision

◆ Skin rashes are more common side effect and to prevent this the best is to avoid sunlight during the mornings from around 10 o'clock to at least 4 o'clock in the evening. Also you can use sunscreen creams or lotion protecting the skin from the sun, avoid wearing see through clothes and also can use umbrella or hat to protect yourself.

◆ Sometimes you may have problems with walking or standing.

◆ It's also noticed that some people may experience fever, throat infections often. This is because of the reduction in the number of certain immune cells in the body.

In case you note that these problems are more then contact your GP or us.

What if I have to become pregnant, as I have heard that this medicine can affect the baby?

Yes that's true. So if you want to become pregnant then let us know, as we need to work with the Obstetrician and then will decide the medications.

This carbamazepine also can reduce the effect of pills so you need to use another method of protection during the period of you taking the medicine.

Drinks can reduce the action of these medications so it's good to cut down drinking. (↑ the sedative effect of the drug).

Is there anything else that you would like to know?

I would be glad to help you.

I'll provide you with the necessary leaflets and information sheets that you can go through.

I appreciate your cooperation. Take care, Bye.

2. ADVICE REGARDING ORAL CONTRACEPTIVE PILLS

Miss Linda is 24-year-old and is interested in pills. Counsel her.

Hello, I am Dr. X Senior House Officer in Gynaecology. How are you feeling today Miss. Linda? As far as I know you had come to us to know about the pills. Well now I am here to tell in detail about the pills. In case you are not able to follow you can stop me at any moment and I will be glad to explain you again. Is that OK?

Before I can actually start off with the actual matter I would like to ask you a few questions. Is that OK with you?

Could you be pregnant?

Do you have high blood pressure?

Have you had any heart problems? Have you had clot in the leg? *Anyone in your* *family has a history of clot in legs? Any liver problems?*

Have you had migraine?

Are you aware of the risks?

Are you aware of the other methods?

Well, the pills contain hormones, which doesn't allow the egg from being released out of the egg-producing gland. Also it makes the normal secretions down below thicker preventing the sperms from entering into the womb.

How do I take these tablets and for how many days do I take them?
The pills should be taken as one every day and at the same timing, for example morning or evening at 8 o'clock so that you will never forget them. Take the pills from the first day of your periods and then continue it as instructed on the cover. It could be 21 tablets with 1-week pill free period or 28 tablets with no pill free period at all. When a packet is done you need to start with the second one from first day of periods.

What if I forget 1 or 2 tablets?
In case you forget to take one tablet then you can take it as soon as you remember but if you have forgotten to take more than that then you need to use extra precaution for the week following that.

What if I want to become pregnant?
You can stop taking the pills and anywhere between few months time you will resume your fertility.

Do I need to take any special precaution during this period of taking pills?
Yes you need to check if you are getting frequent headaches, pain in the leg.

Are there any benefits by taking these pills other than not becoming pregnant?
Yes there are:
◆ The amount of blood loss is less and hence anaemia due to it (Anaemia).

Stop at once if 1) sudden severe chest pain 2) sudden breathlessness with cough & bloody sputum 3) severe calf pain 4) severe stomach pain 5) unusual severe prolonged headache. 6) use condoms during & 7d after taking antibiotics,

◆ The chances of certain breast conditions are rare. (Benign breast conditions) (Breast disease).

◆ The chance of certain diseases of the ovary that is the egg-producing gland is less (Cyst/cancer).

◆ The pain associated with periods is also less (Dysmenorrhoea).

Do these tablets harm in any way?

Well there are a few unwanted effects but these are not necessary to occur in all. I am not trying to scare you. They could be as follows:

◆ Increased chances of acne formation.

• ↑ chances of breast cancer in older women (35-64).

◆ Chances of formation of clot in the leg.

◆ Reduced libido.

◆ Increase in blood pressure.

◆ Migraine.

◆ May some times feel bloated with breast tenderness.

Are there any other tablets available?

Yes the other tablet that is available is POP. But they are less effective than the pills.   Side effect: erratic bleeding, ↑ risk of ectopic pregnancies (pregnancies occuring outside the womb eg in tubes).

Is there anything else that you would like to know?

I would be glad to help you.

I'll provide you with the necessary leaflets and information sheets that you can go through.

I appreciate your co-operation. Take care, Bye.

3. EMERGENCY CONTRACEPTION

Miss Jeena is worried about pregnancy as she had unprotected sex a day back. She wants to know about emergency contraception. Counsel her.

Hello, I am Dr. X Senior House Officer in Obstetrics. How are you feeling today Miss. Jeena? As far as I know you have come to us to know about the emergency contraception. Well now I am here to tell in detail about it. In case you are not able to follow you can stop me at any moment and I will be glad to explain you again. Is that OK?

Before starting with it I would like to ask you a few questions.
Can you tell me when did you have intercourse last?

Can you tell me if you had an unprotected intercourse other than this episode?
Do you use any contraception regularly?
Do you have any discharge from down below?
Do you have migraine or pain in the leg?

There are 2 different methods:
The first one is as tablets, where in we will give you the first dose now and second dose after 12 hours. You will terminate after the second dose.
The second is introducing a coil into the womb and you will subsequently terminate if pregnant. The coil can be used later as a mode of contraception.

Will there be any problem due to this?
Not necessarily, but there may be some amount of bleeding and rarely pain.

Is there anything else that you would like to know?
I would be glad to help you.
I'll provide you with the necessary leaflets and information sheets that you can go through.
I appreciate your cooperation. Take care, Bye.

SECTION 3—COUNSELLING REGARDING DIAGNOSIS

1. ENDOMETRIOSIS

Mrs. Reggie had come with severe bleeding during periods and with dysmenorrhoea. Which was diagnosed as endometriosis. Counsel her regarding this.

Hello I am Dr. X, Senior House Officer in Gynaecology. How are you feeling today Mrs. Reggie?
As far as I know you had come to us with a pain in your tummy and heavy bleeding and after examining you and running a few tests we have diagnosed it as endometriosis and I am here to explain you everything in detail and also to answer all your questions about it and to let you know what we are planning is the best for you? If you are not able to follow you can stop me at any moment. Is that OK?

Normally the womb is lined by certain special cells which are only present within the womb but sometimes they may be present not only inside but also outside the womb such as the tube and egg producing gland as well. Its these cells which cause the normal bleeding during periods and in case of the womb there is a way for the blood to come out but if it's the other sites there is no place for the blood to come out and so they start collecting within the tummy at different sites in the form of small balloon and causes all the problems.

This is not a disease however, though there is no exact and permanent cure available we can treat the symptoms.

◆ Pills are effective during the initial stages.

◆ We can give in the form of tablets that is Danazol.

◆ There are monthly injections which can be given one every month and for 6 months.

◆ There is also a surgery, which we can do, but we cannot remove the entire pockets of the cells by this method.

There are chances of experiencing features similar to menopausal ones but then we will take care of it.

It's very important that you should not become pregnant during this period, as the treatment will affect the baby.

Is there anything else that you would like to know?

I would be glad to help you.

I'll provide you with the necessary leaflets and information sheets that you can go through.

I appreciate your cooperation. Take care, Bye.

2. DIABETES MELLITUS AND ADVICE REGARDING LIFE STYLE CHANGES

Counsel Mr. Atoniette regarding diabetes mellitus and inform about the life style modifications.

Hello I am Dr. X, Senior House Officer in Medicine. How are you feeling today Mr. Atoniette?

As far as I know you had come to us with increased frequency of passing water after examining you and running a few tests we have diagnosed it as diabetes mellitus and I am here to explain you everything in detail and also to answer all your questions about it and to let you know what we are planning is the best for you? If you are not able to follow you can stop me at any moment. Is that OK?

Do you know anything about it?

Well, normally there is a certain amount of sugar present in our blood and all this being controlled by a hormone insulin, sometimes this insulin may reduce in the body and hence the glucose or sugar content increases.

This has no permanent solution but can be corrected by certain changes in our life style and medications or injections.

What lifestyle changes are needed?

◆ First of all your food habits, you have to reduce the intake of red meat and oily food. Reduce the intake of sugar; you can have more of bread and food containing starch. This is in general, however we will refer you to the dietician and he will take care of this.

◆ You need to exercise well which is not only to maintain your health but also to improve the acting of the insulin.

◆ You have to inform the DVLA about the condition

Few important things such as:

◆ Inform your family and colleagues about your condition.

◆ We will have regular follow up and will check your eyes, heart, hands and legs and the functioning of the kidney.

◆ We will inform if there is a change in dosage needed. Do not stop the medication.

◆ Carry the medic alert card with you always. Carry sufficient medicines with you.

◆ We will also inform your GP about this.

Sometimes you may feel very tired, with headache and you may feel irritated, you may sweat excessively with thumping of the heart and sickness and feeling dizzy; this is due to sudden reduction in the glucose. Hence it's always safer to have 1-2 chocolates or candies with you so that you can have them when you get these feelings.

Is there anything else that you would like to know?

I would be glad to help you.

I'll provide you with the necessary leaflets and information sheets that you can go through.

I appreciate your cooperation. Take care, Bye.

3. ASTHMA

Mr. Andrew had come with wheeze and chest tightness. Its been diagnosed as being asthma. Counsel him.

Hello I am Dr. X, Senior House Officer in Medicine. How are you feeling today Mr. Andrew?

As far as I know you had come to us with difficulty in breathing and wheezing and after examining you thoroughly and running a few tests we have diagnosed it as asthma and I am here to explain you everything in detail and also to answer all your questions about it and to let you know what we are planning is the best for you? If you are not able to follow you can stop me at any moment. Is that OK? Do you know any thing about it?

Well, asthma is a common illness, which occurs mainly due to sudden narrowing of the windpipe and this is the pipe through which air comes and goes. This in turn causes all the problems such as tightness and the wheeze also.

Is there any way that I can prevent this from happening?
Yes, there are ways. As you know the actual problem occurs due to allergy to certain things, hence the best is to avoid these allergens. Avoid the following:

◆ Dust.
◆ Smoke and cigarettes.
◆ Gardening and hence the pollen.
◆ Pets if you are allergic to them.
◆ Medicines, which you are allergic to.
◆ Avoid walking in the cold.

The things that you can do are:
◆ Keep your house clean.
◆ Vacuum clean your mattress, pillow, the beddings and the sofa as well as the carpet regularly.
◆ Exercise regularly but do not strain yourself as it can bring about an attack.
◆ Clean your pet regularly if you have one.

Will this alone be sufficient for me by following these advices?
No, it's just not this but there are medications as well that are available. You can take them as inhalers.

I would like to tell in detail about this as well.

There are two types of inhalers in use; a brown-capped one and the other is blue-capped one.

You have to use the medication as prescribed and the blue one is reliever; that is, it relieves the problem so you need to use it when you have an attack. The other one is brown and it is preventer; this is the one, which you need to use regularly everyday as per the prescribed dosage.

I can understand all this but then, what if I get an attack as what had happened this time?

I do understand this very well; just follow these steps:
◆ Do not panic
◆ Sit down on a bed or chair
◆ Relax
◆ Take 1-2 puffs of the blue inhaler, which is very effective in giving you immediate relief

Well I am sure I have answered your questions.
Is there anything else that you would like to know?
I would be glad to help you.
I'll provide you with the necessary leaflets and information sheets that you can go through. I will provide you the information regarding the Asthma Group.
I appreciate your cooperation. Take care, Bye.

4. PARKINSON'S DISEASE

Here is Mr. Dosch who has been diagnosed as having Parkinson's disease. He had come to the OPD with difficulty in walking. Counsel him.

Hello I am Dr. X, Senior House Officer in Medicine. How are you feeling today Mr. Dosch?

As far as I know you had come to us with difficulty in walking and after examining you thoroughly and running the tests we have diagnosed as Parkinson's disease and I will explain you everything in detail and also will answer all your questions about it and will let you know what we are planning is the best for you? If you are not able to follow you can stop me at any moment. Is that OK?

Do you know any thing about it?

First of all I would like to inform that it's not a life threatening condition.

This condition occurs mainly due to absence or deficiency of a chemical substance called Dopamine in the brain. The reason behind this is unknown most of the times. You are going to feel much better as we will give you the chemical substance in the form tablets.

It has been noted that these tablets can cause some amount of sickness and abnormal movement of the legs and hands, in case it's more let us know.

What can be done other than the tablets?

◆ We will refer you to the Physiotherapist and he will teach you few exercises, which will improve your walking and also writing.

◆ We will refer you to the Occupational therapist who will visit your house and will check if anything needs to be changed and then will help you with it.

◆ There are few simple tips that I would like to mention:
Use soft carpets.
Use microwave for cooking.
If using pan turn the handle away from you.

◆ Inform the DVLA.

◆ Restrict heavy exercises.

◆ Avoid clothes with zips and difficult buttons.

◆ The occupational therapist will let you know about fixing rails to the toilet.

◆ Go for flat and soft soled foot wear.

I am worried if this will worsen further?

Mr. Dosch I can understand your worries, but this is a difficult one to answer as it totally depends on how the medicine is going to act on you and how well your body is going to respond to the medicine.

You will be eligible for social security allowance.

Is there anything else that you would like to know?

I would be glad to help you.

I'll provide you with the necessary leaflets and information sheets that you can go through.

I appreciate your cooperation. Take care, Bye.

PLAB-2

5. CERVICAL SMEAR POSITIVE

Mrs. Bennetta is 45-year-old, she had come to get a cervical smear done as routine procedure. Her reports says the smear is positive. Counsel her regarding this.

Hello I am Dr. X, Senior House Officer in Gynaecology. How are you feeling today Mrs. Bennetta?

As far as I know you had come to us to get a routine examination done, one among them was the cervical smear test where in we collected a few cells from the neck of the womb and I am here to explain you everything in detail and also to answer all your questions about it. If you are not able to follow you can stop me at any moment. Is that OK?

The test report says that you have few abnormal cells at the neck of the womb and this is positive.

Oh, does this mean a cancer doctor?

Well Mrs. Bennetta at the moment we cannot tell you, but this not necessarily means it is a cancer but there are high chances that this can turn out to be one. We have to run further tests in order to find out why is this and to know further details about this.

What are you actually planning; I am worried about all this?

We are planning to do another test called the colposcopy where we will use a dye on your neck of womb and then examine thoroughly by using a special instrument and we will take a sample from the abnormal looking site and send it for further tests and when the results are ready we will decide the treatment according to it which may be in the form of heat or cold therapy or a surgery, it could be laser therapy or with current.

We will discuss about it when the results are ready.

I would like to tell at this moment that it is very much necessary to under go these tests as we need to find out at what stage the condition is. That is the reason we need to do the colposcopy.

I hope I am not telling too many things.

I have one more question doctor, could you tell me something about the different stages?

Yes of course I will tell you.

There are 3 stages:

Stage 1 is mild variety where in less than about one-third of the cells are involved.

Stage 2 is a moderate one where in more than one-third of the cells but less than half of them are involved.

Stage 3 is a higher one where in more than half of the cells are involved.

Is there anything else that you would like to know?

I would be glad to help you.

I'll provide you with the necessary leaflets and information sheets that you can go through.

I appreciate your cooperation. Take care, Bye.

SECTION 4—BREAKING BAD NEWS

1. CARCINOMA BREAST IN TERMINAL STAGES

Carry on with breaking the information of cancer breast to Mrs. Joshua, who had come with feeling lump in the right breast.

Hello I am Dr. X, Senior House Officer in Surgery. How are you feeling today Mrs. Joshua?

As far as I know you had come to us with feeling a lump in the right breast and tiredness since a couple of months, for which we did thorough examination and ran a few tests as well.

Before I can proceed, would you like some one else to be here with you?

I am afraid the news is not good.

I am sorry but the results say that you have cancer of the right breast, which has spread to the other parts as well.

Would you like someone else to be here with you?

Pause....

Please take these tissues.

Pause....

Would you like to have some water?

Pause....

Mrs. Joshua, I know that this is very devastating news for you, but we are not going to leave you alone at this point, we will help you as much as possible to take every day as it comes.

PLAB-2

What actually happened doctor, why me?

I am afraid there is no specific cause for this, though its known to run in families. Sometimes it can also occur because of certain hormonal treatment.

Is it in the terminal stage?

I'm afraid the answer is yes as the cancer has spread to involve the lungs and glands in the body as well.

Now how many days do I have with me?

Mrs. Joshua the cancer behaves differently in various patients, moreover the treatment that we offer and the response to the treatment also is different. So there is no answer for this question that I know of. I am sorry.

What can be done for this now?

1. We'll give you pain killers for the pain.
2. We'll refer you to the Oncologist who is a specialist in the treatment of cancer who will decide whether to start you on medicines (Chemotherapy) or to start you on strong X-ray therapy (Radiotherapy)
3. We'll refer you to the Dietician who will take care of your diet and nutrition.
4. We'll have regular follow ups here.
5. We'll also inform your GP
6. We'll provide you the services of Macmillan nurse who are specially trained in taking care of patients with cancer.
7. We'll arrange for the visit of a community nurse.
8. We'll manage bone pain that may arise with strong X-ray therapy.

I know this is very devastating news for you, but then we will try to help you as much as possible.

We are going to work as a multidisciplinary team and all this to make you feel better.

I'll provide you with the necessary details in the form of leaflets. Also I will give you the address of Cancer BACUP, an organization that can help you through your illness and also 24-hour help line.

Is there anything else that you want to ask?

How are you going back home? Is there someone to drive you back?

We'll meet you in the next appointment and you can contact us at any time. Thanks for listening so patiently. Take care and Bye.

2. CARCINOMA CERVIX IN TERMINAL STAGES

Mrs. Vent was admitted with menorrhagia and loss of weight and diagnosed as having cancer cervix. Break this information to her.

Hello I am Dr. X, Senior House Officer in Gynaecology. How are you feeling today Mrs. Vent?

As far as I know you had come to us with excess bleeding from the front passage and tiredness since a couple of months, for which we did thorough examination and ran few tests as well.

Before I can proceed, would you like some one else to be here with you?

I am afraid the news is not good.

I am sorry but the results say that you have cancer of the neck of the womb, which has spread to the other parts as well.

Would you like someone else to be here with you?

Pause....

Please take these tissues.

Pause....

Would you like to have some water?

Pause....

Mrs. Vent, I know that this is very devastating news for you, but we are not going to leave you alone at this point, we will help you as much as possible to take every day as it comes.

What actually happened doctor, why me?
I am afraid there is no specific cause for this, though its known to run in families. Some times it can also occur because of certain hormonal treatment.
It could be due to a viral infection, it's noticed in some women who have multiple partners.

Is it in the terminal stages?
I'm afraid the answer is yes, as the cancer has spread to involve the lungs and glands in the body as well.

Now how many days do I have with me?

Mrs. Vent the cancer behaves differently in various patients, moreover the treatment that we offer and the response to the treatment also varies. So there is no answer for this question that I know of. I am sorry.

What can be done for this now?

1. We'll give you pain killers for the pain.
2. We'll refer you to the Oncologist who is a specialist in the treatment of cancer who will decide whether to start you on medicines (Chemotherapy) or to start you on strong X-ray therapy (Radiotherapy)
3. We'll refer you to the Dietician who will take care of your diet and nutrition.
4. We'll have regular follow ups here.
5. We'll also inform your GP.
6. We'll provide you the services of Macmillan nurse who are specially trained in taking care of patients with cancer.
7. We'll arrange for the visit of a community nurse.
8. We'll manage bone pain that may arise with strong X-ray therapy.

I know this is very devastating news for you, but then we will try to help you as much as possible.

We are going to work as a multidisciplinary team and all this to make you feel better.

I'll provide you with the necessary details in the form of leaflets. Also I will give you the address of Cancer organization that can help you through your illness and also 24-hour help line.

Is there anything else that you want to ask?

How are you going back home? Is there someone to drive you back?

We'll meet you in the next appointment and you can contact us at any time. Take care, Bye.

3. DOWNS SYNDROME

Mr. and Mrs. Ripley had brought their little son pick for general examination as he is not being active since couple of months. He is a year old. It's been diagnosed that he has Downs syndrome. Counsel them.

Hello, I am Dr. X, Senior House Officer in Paediatrics. How are you feeling Mr. and Mrs. Ripley? As you know you had come with little Rick to get him examined, which we have already done and I am afraid that I have got no good news today. I am sorry to tell that he has a condition called Downs syndrome.
Are you aware of this condition?

Well I would like to tell everything in detail to you about this and also to answer your questions about it?

Our body is made up of cells and these have genetic material in them called chromosomes. Normally there are 23 pairs or 46 chromosomes in total. In this condition it is 47 in total. It's the extra chromosome that causes all the problems.

Does this mean he is mentally retarded?
Downs syndrome does not mean mental retardation.
He is a cute kid who is doing well. These babies are usually fun loving and jolly ones who love their parents very much and are very affectionate to them.
They love music and generally are very happy children.
The problem is that the rate at which they develop will be lesser than the other children of the same age group. He may have some problems with his learning.

But what is important is that we will help him to grow to his maximum potential possible and he has that potentiality.

What can be done now?
◆ We will offer services such as support groups, hospital services needed, social and community services. Occupational therapy and physiotherapy.
◆ Special school for his studies.
◆ He'll get Disability Living Allowance.
◆ Downs syndrome organization where you can talk to parents who have child with Downs syndrome.
◆ Regular follow up.

Will he have any other problems because of this problem?
Not necessary that all the babies or children should have but the chances of heart disease is more. Also the chances of skin cancer, problems with hearing and vision. There may be some problems with bowel also.

Is there anything else that you would like to know?

I would be glad to help you.

I'll provide you with the necessary leaflets and information sheets.

I appreciate your cooperation. Take care, Bye.

7 *Clinical Examination*

INTRODUCTION TO EXAMINATION

Here it is a live person who is going to act as a patient. He will mimic the features exactly. The introduction is the same, also include the positioning of the patient. Mention that you will maintain utmost privacy and will request a chaperon.

It is very important to perform all the steps in a systematic fashion without omitting the steps. It is safer to request the patient to do various manoeuvres rather than you getting it done. Take care not to hurt the patient in any way.

This section tests our ability to do systemic examination systematically and professionally at the same time.

MEDICINE

1. RESPIRATORY EXAMINATION

Hello, I'm Dr. ABC, Senior House Officer in Medicine. How are you feeling today Mr. Andrew, I am here to examine your chest. Is that OK? I will be as gentle as possible. For this, I need you to get undressed from the neck to the waist. I will request the presence of a chaperon. If in case there is any discomfort, let me know.

General Examination

First, I'll look into your eyes   ◆   Pallor
Icterus

Now, show your tongue   ◆   Pallor
Cyanosis

Now, show your nails   ◆   Pallor
Icterus
Clubbing

Now, let me see your palm   ◆   Pallor
Icterus

Now, I'll see for oedema in leg

Inspection

Can you stand up for me?
◆ Shape of the chest
◆ Respiratory movement
◆ Respiratory pattern
◆ Respiratory rate
◆ Deformity
◆ Accessory muscles of respiration
◆ Intercostal indrawing
◆ Redness, scar, sinus, visible pulsations, engorged veins.

Palpation

◆ For temperature, tenderness, tracheal position
◆ For respiratory movement
◆ Tactile vocal fremitus
◆ Apex beat

Percussion

◆ Clavicle
◆ Supraclavicle space
◆ Inercostal space
◆ Axillary and infra-axillary region
◆ Suprascapular region
◆ Interscapular region
◆ Subscapular region

Auscultation

For breathsounds and added sounds.

Ideally, I would like to examine the upper respiratory tract, cervical lymph nodes and axillary lymph nodes.

You can get dressed now. Thanks for your co-operation. Thank you doctor.

2. CARDIOVASCULAR SYSTEM

Hello, I'm Dr. ABC, Senior House Officer in Medicine. How are you feeling today? Mr. Jack?I am here to examine your chest. Is that OK? I will be as gentle as possible. For this, I need you to get undressed from the neck to the waist. If in case there is any discomfort, do let me know?

I will be as gentle as possible through out the examination and I will request for the presence of chaperon.

General Examination

First, I'll look into your eyes	◆	Pallor
		Icterus
Now, show your tongue	◆	Pallor
		Cyanosis
Now, show your nails	◆	Pallor
		Icterus
		Clubbing

PLAB-2

Now, let me see your palm   ◆   Pallor

Icterus

Now, I'll examine pulse-rate, rhythm, and character. I'll check JVP.

Inspection

◆ I'll see for any deformed precardium
◆ Any visible pulsations
◆ Apical impulse
◆ Scars, sinus, engorged veins
◆ Respiratory movement and spine.

Palpation

◆ Check temperature, tenderness, trachea.
◆ I'll feel apex beat and for any thrill.
◆ Check parasternal heave.

Auscultation

I'll auscultate in all 4 cardiac auscultatory areas and also base of lung for any crepitation.

Ideally, I would like to examine blood pressure, all peripheral pulses and the liver. You can get dressed now.

Thanks for your co-operation.

Thank you doctor.

3. PER ABDOMEN

Hello, I'm Dr. ABC, Senior House Officer in Medicine. How are you feeling today? Mr. Penny? I am here to examine your tummy. Is that OK? I will be as gentle as possible. For this, I need you to get undressed from the nipple to mid thigh.
I will be as gentle as possible and I will request the presence of a chaperon. If needed in case there is any discomfort, let me know.

General Examination

First, I'll look into your eyes   ◆   Pallor

Icterus

Now, show your tongue	◆ Pallor
	Cyanosis
Now, show your nails	◆ Pallor
	Icterus
	Clubbing
Now, let me see your palm	◆ Pallor
	Icterus

Can you stretch your hands like this in front? (For flapping tremor)

Inspection

Please lie down/sit leaning back. Please bend your knees.

◆ Shape of the abdomen
◆ If corresponding quadrants move equally with respiration
◆ Scars, sinuses
◆ Visible pulsation
◆ Engorged veins
◆ Position of umbilicus.

Palpation

◆ For temperature, tenderness
◆ Superficial palpation from left to right iliac fossa
◆ Guarding and rigidity
◆ Mass
◆ Liver, spleen, kidney
◆ Fluid thrill for ascites
◆ Murphy's sign (positive in acute cholecystitis)
◆ McBurneys tenderness (positive in acute appendicitis)

Percussion

◆ Liver
◆ Ascites.

PLAB-2

Auscultation

◆ For bowel sounds

Ideally, I would also like to examine the axillary and cervical lymph nodes, hernial sites, JVP and I'll do per rectal examination.

You can get dressed now. Thanks for your co-operation. Thank you doctor.

4. CRANIAL NERVE—II-VII

Hello, I am Dr. ABC, Senior House Officer in Medicine. How are you feeling today Mrs. Jose? I am here to examine your face and eyes. I hope you don't mind me. You can stop me if I cause any discomfort.

◆ First, general examination for facial symmetry, ptosis.

II CN

◆ I'll check your eyes and vision now. I'll examine one eye at a time. Can you close your left eye?
1. Count the number of fingers I'm showing. Now repeat with other eye. **(Visual acquity)**
2. Can you read the sentence for me with one eye closed? That's good. Please repeat it with other eye. **(Near vision)**
3. Can you tell me the colour of this pin, one eye at a time? **(Color vision)**
4. Now, I'll close my right eye while you close your left eye. Look through your right eye into my left. I'll wriggle my finger from all directions. Let me know at which point you can see the tip of my finger or if you can't see in any direction. **(Field of vision)**
   That's great. We'll do it with the other eye now.
5. Now, I'll be shining bright light into your eyes while you look straight ahead. It may cause slight discomfort but only for a few seconds. Is that OK?

   Direct
   Indirect ⎤ Light reflex

Ideally, I would have used the Snellens chart for visual acquity and Ishihara's chart for colour vision.

I would also like to do fundoscopy.

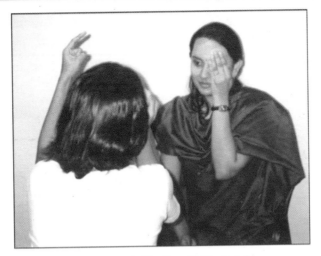

Figure 7.1: Testing field of vision

III, IV, VI CN

◆ Can you follow my finger with your eyes without moving your head? Did you see double vision at any moment?

V CN

◆ I'll touch your face with cotton and when you can feel it let me know. I'll show you once and later we'll examine with closed eyes.
◆ Can you clench your teeth tightly, so that I can feel? Your cheek and forehead?

VII CN

◆ Did you taste your breakfast in the morning?
◆ Can you please show your teeth?
◆ Can you close your eyes tightly, don't allow me to open them.

You have been very co-operative. I appreciate that.
Thank you.
Thank you doctor.

5. CNS EXAMINATION

Examine Sensory and Motor System of Lower Limb.

Hello, I'm Dr. ABC, Senior House Officer in Medicine. How are you feeling today? I'm here to examine the nerves in your leg. For this, I want you to get undressed from below the waist; you can wear your boxers. I'll request the presence of a chaperon.

1. Gait
2. Sensory System

Vibration Sensation

◆ First demonstrate vibration sensation by placing a vibrating 128Hz tuning fork over the sternum. Then, with the patient's eye closed, place the tuning fork over the joints of great toe, ankle joint, medial and lateral malleoli, shin of tibia, knee joint and hip joint one after the other and comparing over both sides simultaneously.

Joint Position Sensation

◆ Demonstrate positions up and down at the metatarsophalangeal joint of great toe, and then with the patient's eye closed, ask him the joint position at MTP joint, ankle joint and knee joint.

Touch Sensation

◆ With the help of wisp of cotton, demonstrate touch sensation over the sternum and then with the patient's eye closed, based upon the dermatomal areas place the cotton wisp to test touch sensation.

Pain Sensation

◆ With a pin, after demonstrating test pain sensation over dermatomal region by asking if it is blunt or sharp end.

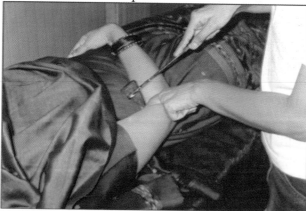

Figure 7.2: Biceps jerk

Temperature Sensation
 ◆ With two test tubes, one containing warm water and the other containing cold water. Check the temperature sensation.

3. Motor System
 ◆ Bulk   —   With measuring tape check the bulk of muscle
 ◆ Power —   Grade it from 0-5
 ◆ Tone   —   Roll the leg over the cot
                         Lift the leg at knee
                         Flex and extend at knee joint
 ◆ Reflexes—   Ankle jerk
                         Knee jerk
                         Plantar jerk
 ◆ Co-ordination of movement
         Heel knee test
         Rombergs test

Thanks for your co-operation. You can get dressed now.
Thanks Doctor.

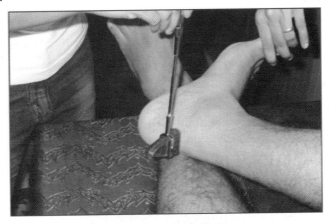

Figure 7.3: Ankle jerk

NOTE:
Examine sensory and motor system of upper limb
The examination is similar to that of lower limb, remember to do biceps, triceps and supinator jerk and for co-ordination its finger-nose test.

ORTHOPAEDICS

1. KNEE EXAMINATION

Hello, I'm Dr. ABC, Senior House Officer in Orthopaedics. How are you Mr. John? I'm here to examine your knee. Is that fine. Please undress from below your thigh. I will be as gentle as possible, in case there is any discomfort let me know. I will request the presence of a chaperon.

Inspection

◆ Deformity–Valgus/varus
◆ Para patellar fullness or if normal
◆ Swelling
◆ Sinus, scar, visible veins, ulcers
◆ Popliteal fossa
◆ Muscle wasting
◆ Gait

Palpation

◆ Temperature
◆ Tenderness
  - Condyles of femur (M + L)
  - Condyles of tibia (M + L)
  - Head of fibula
  - Synovial membrane
  - Patellar surface
  - Medial joint line
  - Lateral joint line
◆ *Massage test*—Empty all fluid from thigh to down the knee. Tap from the side of the patella.
◆ *Patellar tap*—Empty all fluid from thigh to down the knee and push the patella within.

Special Tests

i. *Stress Test*

Lie supine, flex leg at knee for 20°-30°

   Adduct—lateral collateral ligament

 Gently

   Abduct—medial collateral ligament

ii. *Drawer test*

Supine, flex the knee (sit over the foot), clench the fist. Push the leg front, push the leg back. It's for anterior cruciate ligament and posterior cruciate ligament.

iii. *Lachmanns test*

Flex knee for 20°-30°, push femur down and tibia upward and the other way for cruciate ligaments.

iv. *Mc Murray test*

Supine, flex knee for 90°, rotate at the ankle out/in then abduct/adduct at the knee then slowly extend the knee patient will feel pain (out—Medial Meniscus injury: in—Lateral Meniscus injury).

v. *Apleys Grinding test*

Prone position, flex at the knee, compress the tibia over the femur and rotate it internally (L) and externally (M) for menisceal tear.

Movements

◆ Flexion

◆ Extension

Neurovascular Examination

Ideally I would also like to do examination of the hip and the ankle and also limb length measurement.

You have been very co-operative, I appreciate it. Please dress yourself. Thanks Mr. John. Bye

2. HIP EXAMINATION

Hello Mr. Kreig? I am Dr. ABC, Senior House Officer in Orthopaedics. How are you? I am here to examine your hip. Please undress from down, you can wear your underwear. I will request the presence of a chaperon.

I will be as gentle as possible through out the procedure, in case there is any discomfort. Please let me know.

Inspection

◆ Gait
◆ From front I'll see for level of the ASIS
◆ Redness, scars, sinuses, ulcers
◆ Swelling
◆ Muscle wasting
◆ Deformity, limb length discrepancy
◆ Trendelenburg test - Stand on normal leg—Opposite ASIS raises.
　　　　　　　　　　 - Stand on abnormal leg—Opposite ASIS sags

Palpation

◆ Temperature
◆ Tenderness
◆ Greater trochanter
◆ Femoral pulse
◆ Swelling

Special Tests

◆ *Thomas Test* (Fixed Flexion Deformity)
With the patient supine feel for lumbar lordosis. Flex the normal knee and then flex the hip joint at normal side fully, while doing this the abnormal knee will flex. Measure angle between cot and thigh and simultaneously lumbar lordosis disappears.

Movements

◆ Flexion - Extension
◆ Abduction - Adduction
◆ Internal - External rotation

Measurements

◆ Apparent limb length
◆ True limb length (Square the pelvis)

Neurovascular Examination

Ideally I would also like to examine spine, sacroiliac, and knee joint.

Please dress up. Thanks for your co-operation.
Thank you doctor.

3. SPINE

Hello, I am Dr. ABC, Senior House Officer in Orthopaedics. How are you Mr. Cameroon? As far as I know you had come with back pain. Can I examine you? Please undress till waist. I will be as gentle as possible through out the examination.

Inspection

◆ From front—Level of shoulders and thorax
◆ From side—Gibbus, kyphosis, lordosis
◆ From back—Posture, scoliosis, kyphosis
◆ Redness, scars, sinuses, ulcers, visible veins
◆ Swelling
◆ Muscle wasting
◆ Gait

Palpation

◆ Temperature
◆ Tenderness - With the thumb over the spine
              - With the palm over the para-spinal region
              - With the fist give slow beats
◆ Ulcer, swelling

Movement

◆ Flexion—Touch your feet without bending knees
◆ Extension—Bend backwards
◆ Lateral rotation—Move/Bend sideways
◆ Rotation—Sit on the chair, rotate to the Right/Left

Special Tests

1. *SLRT*, Sciatic nerve involvement
   - Supine, raise the leg without flexing (bending the knee) upto 60-120°
   - SLRT is positive if pain is present at less than 45°
2. *Bragards Test*
   - Do SLRT, lower the leg a little less than where you get pain and then dorsiflex at the ankle joint.
3. *Lasegue's Test*
   - Do SLRT, where he gets pain flex knee, flex hip at 90°. Now, extend the knee. If pain occurs, test is positive.
4. *Cruralgia/Femoral Nerve Stress Test*
   - Prone position, flex the knees, as much as possible; if pain is present in anterior thigh it implies test positive.
5. *Sitting Test*—From supine position sit with legs extended on couch. Without supporting with hands.

Neurological Examination

1. Knee jerk
2. Ankle jerk
3. Walk tip toe
   Plantar flexion at ankle
   Sensation in the sole, 5th toe

   S_1

4. Walk on heel
   Dorsiflexion ankle
   Dorsiflexion great toe (EHL)
   Sensation on the dorsum of foot
   At side of leg

   L_5

Ideally I would also like to do PR examination to note the anal sphincter tone, also I would like to examine pelvis.

Thank you Mr. Cameroon for your co-operation.

Thank you doctor.

4. WRIST

Hello, I'm Dr. ABC, Senior House Officer in Orthopaedics. How are you Mrs. Linda? As far as I know you had come following a fall on the right wrist. I'm here to examine your wrist. Is that OK? Can I proceed? I'll be as gentle as possible. Please roll your shirt sleeve up. Are you right handed or left-handed?

Inspection

◆ Swelling
◆ Sinus, ulcer, bruise, scars   } Dorsal + Ventral aspect
◆ Obvious deformity

Palpation

◆ Temperature
◆ Tenderness—Lower end of radius
        Lower end of ulna
        Anatomical snuffbox
◆ Irregularity, deformity
◆ Tap on extended thumb and extended index finger (pain - # scaphoid)
◆ Radial deviation

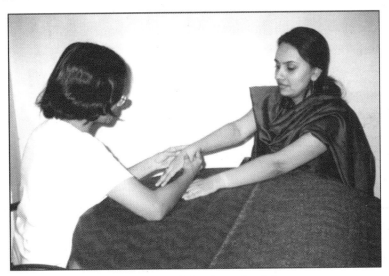

Figure 7.4: Palpation of wrist

Movements

◆ Wrist   - flexion   abduction   supination

               extension   adduction   pronation

◆ Thumb   - flexion   abduction

               extension   adduction

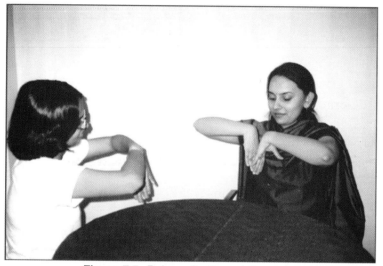

Figure 7.5: Palmar flexion at the wrist

Neurology

◆ Median nerve—Sensation in lateral 3½ fingers, opponens pollices (touch the little finger with the thumb).

◆ Ulnar nerve—Sensation in medial 1½ fingers, hypothenar eminence. Frommets test (hold paper between fingers).

◆ Radial nerve—Sensation in I dorsal interosseous space.

Vascular System

◆ Radial and ulnar artery pulse.

Discuss About MGT

1. Analgesia
2. X-ray wrist AP, lat, oblique view

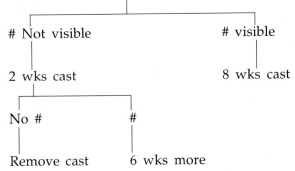

Not visible

2 wks cast

No #   #

Remove cast   6 wks more

visible

8 wks cast

3. Cast from knuckles to below elbow in glass holding position.
4. If no evidence of union even after 8 weeks—surgery
   ORIF + bone grafting.

Complications

1. AVN
2. Nonunion
3. Persistent wrist pain
4. 2° osteoarthritis of the wrist

5. ELBOW

Hello, I am Dr. ABC, Senior House Officer in Orthopaedics. How are you Mrs. Cevin? I am here to examine your elbow. I hope you don't mind. I will be as gentle as possible. Is that fine? Shall I proceed?

Inspection

◆ Deformity
◆ Carrying angle
◆ Limb length discrepancy
◆ Scar, sinus, redness, ulcer
◆ Muscle wasting
◆ Swelling

Palpation

I would be touching your elbow now, please inform me if it's hurting.

◆ Temperature
◆ Tenderness:
  • Supracondylar ridges of humerus
  • ME/LE of humerus
  • Head of radius
  • Olecranon
◆ Medial epicondyl, Lateral epicondyl and Olecranon—Form triangle on flexion and straight line on extension.
◆ Bony irregularities.

Movements

◆ Flexion
◆ Extension
◆ Supination
◆ Pronation

Measurements

Lateral epicondyl—Radius Styloid

Neurovascular Examination

1. Sensory and motor system
2. Radial and brachial artery pulse

Thanks Mrs. Cevin for your co-operation.
Thank you doctor.

6. SHOULDER

Hello, I am Dr. ABC, Senior House Officer in Orthopaedics. How are you Mr. John? I am here to examine your shoulder. Is that OK? Please tell me if it hurts. I will be as gentle as possible. Is that fine? Please undress your upper half of body. I will request the precense of chaperon.

Inspection

◆ Deformity
◆ Swelling
◆ Contour of the shoulder
◆ Muscle wasting
◆ Redness, scars, sinus.

Palpation

◆ Temperature
◆ Tenderness
   • Sternoclavicular joint
   • Clavicle
   • Acromioclavicular joint
   • Acromion
   • Spine of scapula
   • Biceps, deltoid muscle
◆ Swelling, deformity, irregularity.

Movement

◆ Abduction: Steady the scapula with your opposite hand and move the elbow in outwards direction
◆ Adduction: Move towards opposite shoulder
◆ Flexion: From front move it upwards
◆ Extension: Move from back
◆ Place hand behind head—External rotation
◆ Place hand behind back—Internal rotation.

Special Test

◆ Test for painful arc syndrome: Abduct the arm between 40-120°, if pain is present it implies the test is positive.
◆ Flex elbow and against resistance do flexion for bicipital tendonitis.

Measurement

◆ From acromion to the lateral epicondyl—to styloid of radius for limb length.

Neurovascular Examination

1. Sensory and motor system
2. Radial and brachial artery pulse

You can get dressed. Thanks for your co-operation Mr. John

7. RHEUMATOID HAND

Hello, I am Dr. ABC, Senior House Officer in Orthopaedics. How are you Mr. Joe? I am here to examine your hand. Is that OK? I will be as gentle as possible. Is that fine? Please keep your hands over the pillow.

Inspection

- Nails—Splinter haemorrhage, brittle
- Skin—Redness, cyanosis, scars, sinuses
- Subcutaneous nodules
- Deformity of finger
  - DIP Joint
    - Extended—Boutennaires deformity
    - Flexed—Swan neck deformity
  - Thumb
    - Valgus
    - Z deformity
  - Mallet finger
  - Ulnar deviation of the fingers
  - Wrist
    - Z deformity
    - Ulnar deviation
    - Prominence of ulnar/radial styloid

Palpation

- Temperature
- Tenderness—DIP, PIP, MCP, Wrist
- Any nodules, thickening of tendons at the base of fingers while flexing/extending MCP joints.
- Savill pinch test—Pinch for skin over proximal phalanx (If cannot pinch then it is synovitis).

Movement

- ◆ Wrist
  - ◆ Flexion—Place together backs of the hand and raise the hand.
  - ◆ Extension—Prayer position and lower hand
  - ◆ Adduction
  - ◆ Abduction
  - ◆ Supination
  - ◆ Pronation
- ◆ Hand
  - ◆ Grasp my hand
  - ◆ Grip my finger
  - ◆ Pinch your nose
  - ◆ Hold PIP at extension, bend DIP (FDP)
  - ◆ Bend PIP and extension at DIP (FDS)
  - ◆ Flex MCP and extension at PIP and DIP (Lumbricals)
  - ◆ Grasp a paper between fingers (PAD)
  - ◆ Spread your fingers, I'll push with my index finger (DAB)

Neurology

- ◆ Median nerve—Sensation over index finger
- ◆ Radial nerve—Sensation over I dorsal interosseous space
- ◆ Ulnar nerve—Sensation over little finger

Pulse

- ◆ Radial artery
- ◆ Ulnar artery

Ideally, I would also like to examine the:
- ◆ Eyes—Scleritis/Episcleritis
- ◆ Lung—Pleurisy/Effusion/Pulmonary fibrosis
- ◆ Heart—Pericarditis
- ◆ Reflexes
- ◆ Erythema nodosum

Thanks for your co-operation. I'll come back to you again. Take care and Bye.

PLAB-2

SURGERY

1. DIABETIC FOOT EXAMINATION

Hello, I am Dr. ABC, Senior House Officer in Surgery. How are you feeling today, Mrs. Vendall? I am here to examine your legs and foot. For this, I need you to get undressed from below the thighs. I will request the presence of a chaperon. I will be as gentle as possible throughout the procedure. Is that fine? Shall I proceed?

Inspection

◆ I'll see for any ulcers, gangrene, infection in pressure point areas of foot and leg.
◆ Now for any scars and sinuses.
◆ I'll see if there are deformities, swollen joints.
◆ I'll see for muscle wasting.
◆ I'll see for injection sites and lipodystrophy or hypertrophy.

Palpation

◆ Temperature (with back of hand)
◆ Tenderness at joints
◆ Capillary refill
◆ Ulcer/Gangrene
◆ Peripheral pulses
  • Dorsalis pedis artery
  • Posterior tibial artery
  • Popliteal artery
  • Femoral artery

Sensory System Examination

1. *Joint position:* Show up and down position at first IP joint of great toe, ask him to close his eyes and then ask him which is up and which one is down.
2. *Vibration:* Place a vibrating tuning fork over patients sternum and explain him that you will place it over the foot after he closes his eyes and to tell if he can feel the vibration. Repeat it over great toe, medial and lateral malleoli, ankle joint, tibial shaft, tibial tuberosity, knee joint.

3. *Touch sensation*: With cotton wool, examine over segmental areas.
4. *Pain sensation*: With disposable pins with a sharp end and blunt end.
5. *Temperature sensation*: With two containers, one with warm water and the other with cold water.

Motor System

1. Power
2. Tone
3. Reflexes
(Examine both limbs)

Please dress up. Thanks for your co-operation.
Thank the chaperon and also the examiner.

2. PERIPHERAL VASCULAR SYSTEM

Hello, I am Dr. ABC, Senior House Officer in Surgery. Are you Mr. Wendall? How are you? I am here to examine the blood vessels in your legs. Is that fine? Can I proceed? Can you please undress from below your thigh; you can wear your underwear. If there is any discomfort, let me know.

Inspection

◆ Color of the limb
  • Marked pallor—acute ischemia/obstruction
  • Blue/congested—severe ischemia/pregangrenous stage
◆ Nail: transverse ridges, brittle.
◆ Thinning of skin, loss of subcutaneous fat, shiny skin, less hair.
◆ Pressure ulcers over heel, malleoli, below toes, base of the head of metatarsal—site, size, margin, floor, extent, discharge.
◆ Gangrene—Wet or dry, its extent.
◆ Capillary filling time—Can you please raise your legs, now hang your legs down the cot. See if it becomes pale on lifting and then pink later on. It takes more time in ischemia.
  20-30s—Severe ischemia → "BUERGER'S TEST"
◆ Scar, sinuses, varicosities

Palpation

◆ Temperature—Compare both the sides
   Cold + Congested → ischemic limb
◆ Tenderness
◆ Capillary refilling—Press over the nail bed, normally it takes < 2s to come back
   to its colon >if 2s—ischemia
◆ Ulcer
◆ Varicosity

Pulse

◆ Examine both sides
   Dorsalis pedis artery—Over the foot lateral to EHL
   Posterior tibial artery—Behind the medial malleolus
   Popliteal artery—Midline of popliteal fossa
   Femoral artery—Lateral to pubic hair

Auscultation

◆ Femoral artery for bruit

Ideally, I would also like to examine the upper limb, cardiovascular system and take BP.

Also, I would like to examine the sensory and motor system.

Sensory System

◆ Sensation in both the legs
   • Touch
   • Pain/pressure

Please dress up. Thanks for your co-operation.

Thank you doctor

3. THYROID EXAMINATION

Hello, I am Dr. ABC, Senior House Officer in Surgery. How are you Mr. Kennedy? I am here to examine your neck. I will be as gentle as possible. Is that fine? Can I proceed? Can you please undress till your nipple?

General Examination

- ◆ Nails   — Pallor, clubbing, cyanosis
- ◆ Hands   — Tremor, sweating, warmth
- ◆ Pulse   — Rate, rhythm
- ◆ Tongue — Tremor
- ◆ Leg   — Pretibial myxoedema

Inspection

- ◆ Any obvious swelling
- ◆ Please take a sip of water, don't swallow. Please swallow when I ask you to (see for the swelling/lump).
- ◆ Please stick your tongue out (see for any swelling).
- ◆ Scar, sinuses, redness, skin changes.
- ◆ Dilated veins.
- ◆ Visible pulsation.

Palpation

I am going to touch your neck now. Please tell me, in case you are having any discomfort. Fine.

- ◆ Position of trachea.
- ◆ Go behind the patient and palpate for the thyroid lobes first and then the isthmus, palpate once asking patient to swallow.
- ◆ Laheys method from front, push the gland from left to right to palpate right side and vise versa.
- ◆ Swelling—Size, shape, surface, consistency, diffusely smooth or nodular fixity, mobility, tenderness.
- ◆ Feel for the lower border.
- ◆ Lymph nodes
  Submental, submandibular, JDLN, cervical lymph nodes. supraclavicular lymph nodes.

Percussion

If retrosternal extension present, then it will be dull on percussing over sternum.

PLAB-2

Auscultation

For bruit over the upper lobe.

Pulse

Carotid artery.

Eye

◆ Exophthalmos—From behind lift the patients head slowly and see.
◆ Extra-ocular movements.
◆ Lid lag.

Reflex

◆ Ankle jerk

Please dress up. Thanks for your co-operation.
Thank you doctor.

8 Basic Skills

1. CARDIOPULMONARY RESUSCITATION (ADULT)

Good Morning, I am Dr. ABC.

1. Is it safe for me to approach the patient?
2. Is the patient safe? Is the environment safe?
3. Has the patient sustained any injury?
    i. Hello! Hello! Can you hear me? Can you hear me?
    ii. Help. Help. Help.
    iii. I'll do head tilt, chin lift and see for any foreign body.
    iv. Look, listen and feel for breath sounds for 10 seconds. Look at the chest for respiratory movements, listen for breath sounds from nose and feel for air on my cheek.
    v. I'll dial 999, "Hello, I am Dr. ABC, calling from GMC, I Floor, Great Portland Street, London. There is an adult male patient unconscious here. Please activate the adult resuscitation team. Can you repeat the address? Thank you."
    vi. Head tilt, chin lift, pinch nose. I'll give 2 rescue breaths.
    vii. I'll feel for carotid pulse for 10 seconds.
    viii. With right middle finger, I will trace the rib border and with the index finger above it. Place heel of one hand just above, lock other hand, start compression at the rate of 15 : 2.

2. CARDIOPULMONARY RESUSCITATION (PAEDIATRIC)

Good Morning, I am Dr. ABC.

1. Is it safe for me to approach the patient?
2. Is the patient safe? Is the environment safe?

PLAB-2

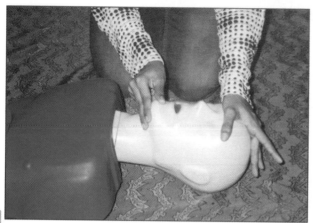

Figure 8.1: Head tilt and chin lift to check for foreign body

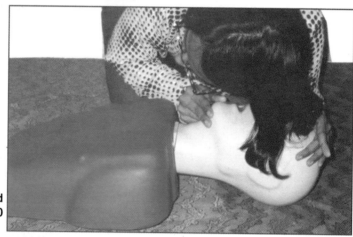

Figure 8.2: Look, listen and feel for breath sounds for 10 seconds

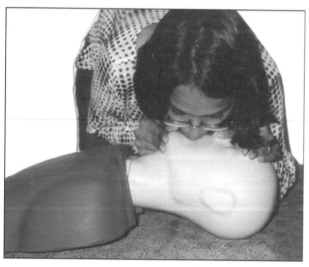

Figure 8.3: Mouth-to-mouth respiration

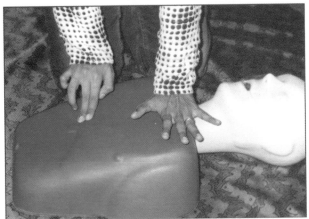

Figure 8.4: Chest compression at a rate of 15 : 2
(compression : respiration)

3. Has the patient sustained any injury?

 i. Hello! Hello! Can you hear me?

 ii. Help. Help. Help.

 iii. I'll do chin lift, moderate head tilt and look, listen and feel for respiratory movements and breath sounds for 10 seconds. Remove foreign body, if present.

 iv. I'll give two rescue breaths.

 v. I'll check carotid pulsation for 10 seconds.

 vi. I'll place one hand over the right index finger after tracing the rib border and give compression and rescue breath at ratio of 5 : 1.

 vii. Do this for one full minute, then go ring 999, "Hello, I'm Dr. ABC, calling from GMC Venue, I Floor, Great Portland Street, London. There is a paediatric male patient who has collapsed. Please activate the paediatric resuscitation team. Can you repeat the address? Thank you."

 viii. I'll give two rescue breaths.

 ix. With right index finger, I'll trace the rib border and place heel of one hand above this and give compression at the rate of 5 : 1.

 x. Now, I'll continue compression and respiration at a rate of 5 : 1.

Thank You.

3. PRIMARY SURVEY

I'll alert the trauma team first. Assuming that I'm gloved, gowned and goggled. I'll take an ATLS walk and greet the patient if he is conscious and obtain permission to examine him.

"Since you have sustained a major injury, I have to first stabilize your neck and put a collar".

i. AIRWAY

   i. I'll do manual stabilization by holding shoulders and supporting the head with my forearm.
   ii. I'll ask, "How are you? Are you fine?" If he answers, it implies that airway is patent.
   iii. I'll request the nurse to swap hands and I will see for the airway.
   iv. I'll do chin lift/jaw thrust to see if there is any obstruction, foreign body, bleeding in the mouth and I'll remove it.
   v. I'll do suction and later I'll place oral airway or nasopharyngeal airway. If not, the definitive management is endotracheal intubation.
   vi. I'll give 100% oxygen via a facemask.
   vii. I'll examine the neck to see if there are any engorged veins, injury and tracheal shift.
   viii. Now, I'll put the cervical collar, place 2 sandbags and put 2 tapes one over forehead and the other one over the chin, i.e. triple immobilization.
   ix. I'll request the nurse to connect 3 monitors:
   - ECG
   - Pulsoximeter
   - BP Monitor

ii. BREATHING

- I'll inspect the patient's face for cyanosis, chest for injury, respiratory movement, and bleeding, accessory muscles of respiration.
- I'll palpate for respiratory movements.
- I'll percuss for dullness or increased resonance.
- I'll auscultate for breath sounds and if any added sounds present.

i. *Pneumothorax*—I'll insert wide bore needle into II intercostal space, mid clavicular line on the affected side and leave it until I put a chest drain or connect it to underwater seal drain.

ii. *Flail chest*—I'll give analgesia to patient, oxygen and I'll do strapping of chest.

iii. *Haemothorax*—Put IV cannula in both hands and at the end of the procedure chest drain is put in V intercostal space in mid axillary line on the affected side.

iv. *Cardiac tamponode*—I'll put a long needle in the IV intercostal space, left to xiphisternum towards left scapula while monitoring the ECG. Leave it and later insert a catheter and remove the needle.

iii. CIRCULATION

◆ I'll have a check on pulse, BP, respiratory rate, pulse pressure, O₂ saturation.

◆ I'll look for change of colour of face (pale) and if periphery is cold.

◆ I'll put 2 IV cannula's one in each forearm.

◆ I'll obtain blood for investigation – Full blood count, urea and electrolyte, blood glucose, blood grouping and typing, cross matching 6 U and I'll request for 2 U of universal blood and 4 U of group specific blood.

◆ I'll start 2L of warm Hartmann's solution. If external bleeding seen, I'll control it with pressure.

◆ For internal bleeding:

i. *Abdomen*—I'll see if there is any distension, injury, bruise, palpate for guarding and rigidity, percuss for dullness, auscultate bowel sound. If bleeding suspected, then I'll seek help from my surgery colleague for DPL/Laparotomy after an USG.

ii. *Pelvis*—I'll examine the pelvis for injury, bleeding, deformity, and blood in external urethral meatus. I'll do spring test only once and inform my orthopaedic colleague to help, if external fixator is needed.

iii. *Thigh and leg*—I'll inspect the thigh and leg for any bleeding, injury, deformity, fracture chips, if seen. I'll feel for any deformity and if fracture suspected I'll put a splint, check pulse and later get an X-ray done. I'll request my orthopaedic colleague so as to help in managing further.

iv. DISABILITY

◆ I'll see the pupil and for reaction to light. I'll see if he is alert. I'll see if he responds to verbal comment (How are you? Are you alright?). I'll see if he responds to pain.

v. EXPOSURE

◆ I'll see to it that I perform the survey by exposing the patient, i.e. by removing the clothes and preventing hypothermia by covering with blanket.

ADJUNCTS

1. ECG, pulsoximetry, BP
2. Three primary X-rays—Chest X-ray; cervical spine X-ray (Lateral); Pelvis X-ray (AP)
3. Ultrasound; DPL
4. Nasogastric intubation, urinary catheter.

4. SECONDARY SURVEY

I'll first greet the patient, take his permission for examination. Assuming that primary survey has been done, airway secure and neck stabilized, patient exposed completely and hypothermia prevented and connected to the monitor. After taking universal precautions. I'll proceed.

◆ I'll take history from the patient; ideally I would like to take a detailed history.
   A—If he is **allergic** to anything.
   M—If he is on any **medication**.
   P—Any relevant **past medical conditions**.
   L—When did he have his **last meal**?
   E—**Events** related to the injury.

◆ Now, I'll start with head to toe examination.
   i. *Scalp*—I'll see for any laceration, depressed #, wound, bruise and bleeding.
   ii. *Mastoid*—For bruise (Battles sign).
   iii. *Ear*—I'll see for foreign body, bleeding and CSF otorrhoea. Ideally I'll do otoscopy.
   iv. *Forehead*—For fracture, bruise, bleeding.

  v. *Eyes*—For discolouration, bruise around eyes (Raccoons sign); subconjunctival haemorrhage, foreign body, injury to cornea, sclera, lens. Ideally, I'll do fundoscopy.

 vi. *Nose*—For foreign body, bleeding, CSF rhinorrhoea, fracture, septal haematoma.

vii. *Oral cavity*—For bleeding, foreign body, fracture, palate, loose tooth.

viii. *Mandible*—For dislocation.

 ix. *Neck*—For wound, bleeding, tracheal shift, engorged veins, tenderness, carotid pulse. (After requesting the patient to not to move his neck. I'll open the hard collar and have a quick look).

  x. *Chest*
   - Inspection—Bruise, injury, respiratory rate, movement.
   - Palpation—Tender clavicle, sternum, chest movement
   - Percussion—Dullness/Resonance
   - Auscultation—Breath sounds and heart sounds.

 xi. *Abdomen*
   - Inspection—For distension, bleeding, bruise, injury
   - Palpation—Tenderness, guarding, rigidity
   - Percussion—Dullness
   - Auscultation—Bowel sounds

xii. *Pelvis*—I'll see X-ray pelvis and manage accordingly.

xiii. I'll look for bones for fracture, any tears or cuts.

xiv. Ideally I'll open the bandage and examine for: (if there are any)
   - Injury, bleeding, bruise, deformity
   - Temperature, tenderness
   - Movement and tests
   - I'll take X-ray at the end of the procedure and manage accordingly.

 xv. I'll ask him:
   - Lift your leg, move your knee, bend at ankle
   - Lift your arm, bend at elbow, move your wrist

xvi. I'll do neurological examination
   - GCS
   - Cranial nerve examination
   - Motor and sensory system, power, tone and reflexes

xvii. I'll complete by doing P.R. examination and putting NGT and urinary catheter, if needed.

5. EXAMINE COMATOSE/UNCONSCIOUS PATIENT

Assuming that airway, breathing and circulation has been secured and cervical spine being stabilized, oxygen given and venous access gained, I would give 50 ml of 50% dextrose if blood glucose is < 5 mm/L.

I will check the following:

1. Signs of injury over the head, lacerations, bleeding, bruise, fracture.
2. I'll examine the neck to see, if there is stiffness. (Not if he has sustained injury to the neck).
3. Foreign body, bleeding or CSF in ear, nose, mouth.
4. Haemorrhage in eye, pupillary size.
5. I'll smell for ketones, drugs, alcohol.
6. I'll see the wallet for any drugs, medic alert card and smell for alcohol.
7. I'll see the arm, forearm for any tell tale signs of drug abuse.
8. Check for allergy band.
9. I'll check over the forearm and thigh for injection marks for diabetes.
10. I'll see for skin rashes on the body, signs of injury, bleeding, cyanosis, pallor.
11. I'll examine heart and lungs (murmurs, breath sounds, added sounds).
12. Auscultate the abdomen for bowel sounds and see for guarding and rigidity.
13. I would like to do otoscopy and fundoscopy.
14. I'll do GCS scoring.

    i. Can you hear me?
    (Verbal)

    Scoring from 5
    - Responds
    - Confused reply
    - Inappropriate reply
    - Incomprehensive reply
    - No response

    ii. Can you lift your hand?
    (Motor)

    Scoring from 6
    - Lifts
    - Localizes to pain
    - Withdraws to pain
    - Flexes to pain
    - Extends to pain
    - No response

iii. Can you open your eyes?
    (Eyes)

Scoring from 4
- Opens spontaneously
- Opens to verbal stimulus
- Opens to painful stimulus
- No response

15. I'll do complete neurological examination.
16. I'll obtain history from the patient's relative and paramedics.

6. GLASGOW COMA SCALE (GCS) AND NEUROLOGICAL EXAMINATION

1. Hello, can you hear me, are you alright? [5]
2. I'll look at the eyes for eye opening [4]
3. Can you lift your hand up? [6]
4. I'll give painful stimulus and see patient's response for – eyes, motor and also verbal response.
   I'll pinch or press over sternum and note
   - Sound
   - Eye
   - Movement
5. I'll do the neurological examination
   i. First motor system
   - Tone
     Lower limb – Roll leg/lift below knee/flex and extend knee
     Upper limb – Move wrist/move at elbow
   - Bulk—On inspection appears to be normal, but I will examine using a measuring tape.
   - Power – I'm unable to do, as he is unconscious.
   - Reflexes.
   ii. Sensory examination—I'm unable to do as patient is unconscious.
   iii. Cranial nerve examination—I can only do this, examine his eyes for:
   - Pupil size
   - Reaction to light
   - Direct and indirect light reflex

7. COGNITIVE STATE EXAMINATION

1. How are you feeling Mr. Hudson?

    NOTE: Appearance   -   Whether dressed cleanly

    -    Unkempt

    Behaviour   -   Low

    -    Anxious

    Eye contact

    Mood   -   Low

    -    Normal

    -    High

    Speech

2. You seem to be low?

    Are your always like this?

    Does your mind change a lot?

    Do you have the energy to do things?

    What do you feel the future holds for you?

3. What's going on in your mind?

4. Do you feel someone's trying to steal your thoughts or insert into your mind?

5. Do you feel someone's trying to harm you?

6. Can you tell me the numbers from 20 to 1?

7. I'll tell an address, repeat it after me.   **Concentration**

    I Floor, GMC, Great Portland Street, London.

8. Can you tell me when was the I World War? **(Memory)**

9. Tell me the name of this city and country? Tell me today's date, month and year. **(Orientation)**

10. Do you think you are not feeling fine? Do you feel you need treatment? (Insight)

    NOTE: • ABCDE – HI – MS – O

    • Appearance

    • Behaviour

    • Concentration

    • Delusion

    • Emotion/Eye contact

    • Hallucination

- Illusion/Insight
- Memory
     Short-term
     Long-term
- Speech
- Orientation

8. MMSE

Hello Mr. Hevyner. I am Dr. ABC; Senior House Officer in Psychiatry. How are you feeling? I am here to have a small talk with you during which I would be asking you a couple of questions. Some of them may sound to be silly but it is relevant here. Is that OK?

  i. Orientation to time – [5]
     Can you tell me today's date, day, month, year and season?
 ii. Orientation to place – [5]
     Can you tell me which city is this, the street, building, floor and country we are in?
iii. Attention and calculation – [5]
     Spell the word 'WORLD' backwards (DLROW)
     OR
     Subtract 7 from 100, 5 times consecutively
     [100 - 7= 93 – 86 – 79 – 72 – 65]
 iv. Registration – [3]
     Can you repeat the 3 words that I'm going to say now – apple, biscuit and chocolate?
  v. Three stage command – [3]
     Take this paper in your right hand, fold it into half and put it on the floor.
 vi. Language, naming – [2]
     I'll show you 2 objects, tell me what it is – hair, chair
vii. Repeating – [1]
     Can you repeat this please!
     "No ifs, ands or buts"
viii. Recall – [3]
     Can you repeat those three words that I have already said [a, b, c]?

ix. Reading – [1]

Can you do what's written on the card "CLOSE YOUR EYES"?

x. Writing - [1]

Can you write a complete sentence?

xi. Construction – [1]

Can you copy this?

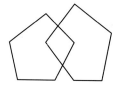

TOTAL SCORE - 30

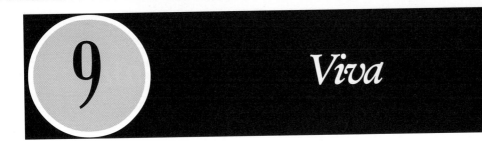

Viva

This is one section of PLAB-2 exams that may be asked sometimes. The topics commonly asked are in the OHCM.

The commonly asked ones are:
1. Management of MI
2. Management of CCF
3. Management of DKA
4. Management of Status Epilepticus
5. Management of Acute Severe Asthma
6. Management of PCT Poisoning (Paracetamol)

One has to be very much thorough with the symptoms and signs, the investigations and treatment as well as the complications of these conditions.

NOTE:
1. An ECG of M.I. can be given in a viva station of M.I.
2. An X-ray, chest (pneumonia) can be given for a DKA station.
3. A graph may be provided for a PCT poisoning viva station.

HISTORY TAKING

1. WEIGHT GAIN

Hello, I am Dr. ABC, Senior House Officer in Medicine, how are you feeling Mrs. Christine. As far as I know you have come here with concerns of having put on weight. I would like to ask you a few questions regarding this to find out what's causing this. Is that OK?

◆ What was your weight previously? What is it now? In how many days has your weight increased?

◆ Do your pee frequently? Any problem with your waterworks? Do you feel tired often? **(Diabetes)**

◆ What about your bowel habits? Do you feel any lump in the throat? Any difficulty in swallowing food?

   Do you dislike cold? **(Hypothyroidism)**

◆ What about your mood? What about your appetite and food habits? What do you feel about the future? **(Depression)**

◆ What about your periods? Are they regular?
   Do you have heavy periods or light ones? Are you on any medications? **(Cushing's disease)**

◆ Do you get headache often? Any increased hair growth on the face? How many children do you have? **(PCOD and brain tumours)**

◆ Are you on HRT or pills now? Do you have any other illness?

◆ Do you smoke, drink or use drugs?

◆ What about your blood pressure and blood sugar?

◆ Does anyone else in your family have similar problems?

◆ Are you on any medication? Are you allergic to anything?

Is there anything else that you would like to tell me?

I appreciate your co-operation. Take care and bye.

2. HOARSENESS OF VOICE

Hello, Mr. Andrew Hugh. I am Dr. ABC, Senior House Officer in Accident and Emergency. Well, you seemed to be having trouble with your voice isn't it? Can I ask you a few questions to find out what is causing this?

◆ Since when are you having this problem?

   Did it start all of a sudden or has been building gradually?

   Does anything worsen it? What makes you feel better?

◆ Do you have running temperature? Any pain in the throat?

   Do you have difficulty in swallowing?

   How about a cough or cold? **(Infective laryngitis)**

   Did you take part in a mass meeting or a football match and played a part as a cheering person? **(Traumatic laryngitis)**

◆ Do you have any concerns about your weight and appetite?

   Did you notice any glands in your body? **(Cancer larynx)**

◆ Did you sustain a trauma to the neck?

◆ Do you have any other medical or surgical illness?

◆ Do you smoke, drink or use recreational drugs? What about your blood pressure and blood sugar?

◆ Does anyone else in your family have similar problems?

◆ Are you on any medication? Are you allergic to anything?

   Is there anything else that you would like to tell me?

   I appreciate your co-operation. Take care and bye.

3. TOE JOINT PAIN

DD's   — Gout

         — Pseudogout

         — Rheumatoid arthritis

         — Trauma

         — SLE

PLAB-2

— Reiter's disease

— Connective tissue disorders

4. EAR PAIN

DD's — Otitis externa

— Otitis media

— Furruncle

— Trauma

— Barotrauma

— Cervical spondylosis

— Wax

— Foreign body

5. SUICIDE

Hello Mrs. Jovit. How are you feeling now? I am Dr. XYZ, Senior House Officer in Psychiatry. I would like to have a small talk with you if you don't mind. I assure you it will be confidential.

◆ What actually happened?

What's going on in your mind now?

When and where did you take the tablets?

Did you drink before this? Did you write any letter prior to this?

Was there someone else with you?

Did you give a party to your loved ones before this act?

How long have you been planning this?

How did you collect the tablets?

How did the medical staff get to know?

Have you attempted suicide before?

How do you feel now that you are alive? Do you feel like repeating it again?

What do you feel the future has in store for you?

Are you able to sleep well and eat well?

Do you have the energy to do your activities?

◆ Any other medical or psychiatric illness?

◆ Do you smoke, drink or use drugs? What about your blood pressure and blood sugar?

◆ What about your married life, your family, work?
◆ Does anyone else in your family have similar problems?
   Is there anything else that you would like to tell me?

   You have been very co-operative.
   I will come back to you later. Thanks.

6. PANIC ATTACKS

Hello Mrs. Friedman, I am Dr. XYZ, Senior House Officer in Psychiatry. As far as I know you have come with certain complaints. I need to ask you a few questions regarding this to find out what is causing this?
◆ What actually is happening to you?
   Since when are you having this feeling?
   How did it start?
◆ What worsens it? What makes you feel better?
   Is your day-to-day work affected by this?
◆ During the attack, do you feel that your mouth dries, you get sick, feel butterflies in the stomach, have loose stools?
◆ Do you feel tightness in the chest, suffocation?
◆ Does your heart pound excessively and sweat more?
◆ Do you feel dizzy and have tremors? Do you feel something bad is going to happen?
◆ Do you feel your weight has changed? Any mood changes? **(Thyrotoxicosis)**
◆ Do you pee frequently, feel more thirsty and eat more? **(Diabetes)**
◆ Do you get headache frequently? **(Phaeochromocytoma)**
◆ Have you any other medical or psychiatric illness?
◆ Do you smoke, drink or use drugs? What about your blood pressure and blood sugar?
◆ Do you take excess coffee, tea? Do you have a lot of stress and tension about your work, family or finance? What about your partner and sexual life?
◆ Does anyone else in your family have similar problems?
◆ Are you on any medication? Are you allergic to anything?

Is there anything else that you would like to tell me? I appreciate your co-operation. Thanks

7. RISK FACTORS FOR TIA

Mrs. Amanda has come with numbness in her right little finger. Take relevant history from her and find out if there are any risk factors for TIA.

Hello, I am Dr.X Senior House Officer in medicine. How are you feeling Mrs. Amanda? As far as I know you had come to us with numbness in your little finger and I would like to ask you a few questions regarding it, to find out what the cause is. Is that OK with you?

It will last for a few minutes only.

◆ Where did the numbness start first?

Was it sudden or has it been occurring since a few days?

Is it present continuously or does it just come and go?

Does it spread anywhere else or to the other parts of the body?

What worsens it?

What makes you feel better?

How long does it last?

Do you feel any other abnormal sensations?

Have you had any problems with speaking, swallowing food, chewing?

Do you have blurring of vision, weakness in any part of the body?

Have you had black outs or dizziness?

◆ Have you had similar experience previously? Any other medical illness or any surgeries that you had undergone?

◆ Have you had any heart problems, high blood pressure, and stroke?

◆ Have you had any disease of the blood vessels?

◆ Did you travel on air recently?

Were you admitted in a hospital for long?

Did you have pain in your leg and were you diagnosed as having clot in the leg or lung?

◆ Are you on pills or any hormone therapy?

◆ Are you on blood thinners?

◆ Have you checked your blood sugar and cholesterol levels?

◆ Did anyone in your family have similar problems, any one with stroke or any heart disease, diabetes?

Did anyone sustain a sudden death in your family?

◆ Do you smoke, drink or use any recreational drugs?

◆ Are you on any medication?

◆ Are you allergic to anything?

Is there anything else that you would like to tell me?

I appreciate your co-operation; I will come back to you later. Take care and thanks.

COUNSELLING

1. DYSMENORRHOEA

Obtain history and counsel.

Hello, I am Dr. ABC, Senior House Officer in Obstetrics. How are you feeling Mrs. Lisa? As far as I know you had come here with pain in your tummy during periods isn't it? I would like to ask you a few questions regarding this. Is that OK?

◆ Since when are you having this pain? Does it come every month?

Where exactly is it? Can you describe this?

How long does it last?

What worsens it? What makes you feel better?

Does the pain start along with your periods? When does it stop?

What about your periods? Are they regular? Are they heavy or light?

When was your last period?

Could you be pregnant?

◆ Do you have any problem with your bowel or waterworks?

◆ Do you have pain during intercourse? **(Endometriosis)**

◆ Do you bleed during intercourse? **(Cervical cause)**

◆ Do you have running temperature?

Do you have any discharge down? **(PID)**

◆ Do you feel any mass or lump in your tummy? **(Fibroid)**

◆ Do you use any contraceptive methods?

◆ Do you have any other medical or psychiatric illness?

◆ Do you smoke, drink or use drugs? What about your blood pressure and blood sugar?

◆ Anyone else in your family with painful periods?

◆ Are you on any medication? Are you allergic to anything?

Mrs. Lisa, this is a condition called dysmenorrhoea, i.e. painful periods. It is quite a common condition and we can treat it as well.

What is important is to relax, take rest, exercise, have fun and forget about the pain. This does workout for a few of them.

In case it does not work out, there are:

◆ Simple analgesics like PCT.

◆ NSAIDs—Mefanamic acid and its quite effective.

◆ OCP—They reduce the pain and also the periods will be lighter.

◆ Antispasmodics

◆ Women after childbirth have lesser period's pain.

Thanks and Bye.

2. MENORRHAGIA

Hello, I am Dr. ABC, Senior House Officer in Obstetrics. How are you feeling Mrs. Deni? I would like to ask you a few questions regarding your problem. Is that OK?

◆ Since when are you having this problem? How many days does it last for?
Is it heavy? Do you pass clots?
How many pads do you change?
When was your last period? Have your periods been regular previously?

◆ Could you be pregnant? **(Abortion, ectopic pregnancy)**

◆ Do you have pain in the tummy? Do you feel any lump/mass in your tummy?
Do you have burning waterworks?
Do you pee frequently? **(Fibroid)**

◆ Are you using any contraception? **(Coil)**

◆ Do you feel any hot flushes, night sweats, and mood swings, bloating? **(Menopause)**

◆ Do you dislike cold? Do you feel you have put on weight and you have problems with opening bowel? **(Hypothyroidism)**

◆ Do you have any bleeding disease?

◆ Do you feel you have lost weight and appetite?
Do you feel glands in your body? **(Cancer cervix, cancer endometrium)**

Well Mrs. XYZ, we need to perform a few tests like blood tests, test your water, TV scan through tummy and also through the front passage and special X-rays. Initially, we will give you medications –

◆ Tranexemic acid as it reduces bleeding
◆ Combined pills
◆ Mirena coil is a good option, both to prevent pregnancy and also for the bleeding.
◆ Finally, there are surgeries such as —
    ◆ Microwave endometrial resection/ablation
    ◆ Hysterectomy.

3. ANTEPARTUM HAEMORRHAGE

Hello, I am Dr. ABC, Senior House Officer in Obstetrics. How are you feeling Mrs. Janet? I would like to ask you a few questions regarding your problem. Is that OK?

◆ How many months pregnant are you?
    Do you have pain in the tummy?
    Since when are you bleeding? Is it in the form of a spot or more?
    Is it painful/painless?
    Does your tummy feel hard? Can you feel the baby move?
    Did you sustain trauma?
    Do you have any itching, rashes or discharge down below?
    Did you bleed when you had intercourse?
    Is this the first time?
    What about your previous pregnancies?
    Did you have any problem during antenatal period?
    Have you got a scan done? Was it normal?
    Are you using blood thinners?

Well, this bleeding could be due to:

◆ The afterbirth lying at lower level. **(Placenta praevia)**
◆ Afterbirth has separated slightly from the inner lining of the womb **(Abruptio placenta)**

We will have to run a few tests to confirm it. The best would be to admit you as:

◆ You need a lot of rest and monitoring.

◆ We need to run a few tests like blood tests, TV scan, urine test, and clotting profile.

◆ We need to monitor your baby by CTG – i.e., trace of the baby.

◆ Then, our consultant will decide whether to send you home or to keep you back.

4. PAIN RELIEF IN PREGNANCY

Hello, I am Dr. ABC, Senior House Officer in Obstetrics. How are you feeling Mrs. Johann? As far as I know you have come here to know about pain relief in pregnancy is not it? Well, I will explain everything in detail.

◆ *Why does this pain occur?*

It is mainly because of tightening of the muscles in the womb and its normal during pregnancy as this helps the baby to come out of the womb.

1. Your partner will be here with you; also your mother or sister will be here. Most of the time, this itself is helpful, as the *moral support* will favour you to reduce the pain.

2. *Entonox:* This is gas; it is a mixture of O_2 and laughing gas N_2O. This gives pain relief without oversleeping, takes 30 – 40s to start acting. So, when the contraction starts you can use this gas that will be delivered through a mask, and by the time the pain reaches its peak, the gas would have already started to act and so reduces pain.

Sometimes, it can however cause dry mouth, sickness. We will give you water in the form of sips.

3. We can give you injection *pethidine* into your buttocks, the effect of which will last for 1½ - 3 hours. We will stop it 2-3 hours before the baby is delivered as it can cause breathing problems in the baby. You can take it by yourself as patient controlled analgesia.

4. *Epidural:* It is injection given to the back and we will insert a thin tube and leave it there, whenever pain relief is needed we can give the medicine through this tube itself. Since the chance of BP to fall is there, we will give fluids into your vein. Top up can be done as and when needed. You can move around freely.

I hope I have answered everything. Take care and see you soon. Bye

5. LOW BACK PAIN

Hello, Mr. Richard, how are you feeling? I am Dr. ABC, Senior House Officer in Orthopaedics? As far as I know you have come here with problems in your back and sore back.

Well, we need to run a few tests to see if we can find out what is causing it.
◆ Like blood test, test of water, X-ray, CT scan and MRI if needed.

Coming to the treatment aspect –
1. Get on with your activities as in within the limits of pain.
2. You can take rest for a few hours, but get yourself moving after that.
3. We will provide you with the necessary painkillers, initially PCT but incase pain does not subside, can even give naproxen – NSAID
4. Can keep warm towel or hot water bag over the back, it surely will reduce the soreness.
5. Swimming in warm water is beneficial.
6. It is important that you exercise but within the pain limits.
   ◆ Bend front and back
   ◆ Move your body to right and left without bending your knees.
   ◆ Twist to right and left.
7. We'll refer you to the physiotherapist who will train you on how to exercise and strengthen the muscle, how to maintain a posture and how to lift things.
8. Avoid lifting heavy weight.
9. Can lie down on flat surface, can keep wooden board over the mattress to get the hard platform for you to sleep on.
10. Lying down straight is very important.

Is there anything else that you want to know. I will come back to you. Take care and bye.

6. PID

Hello, Mrs. XYZ, how are you feeling? I am Dr. ABC, Senior House Officer in Gynaecology. As far as I know you are here to know regarding the cause for discharge from your front passage. Am I right?

Well, at the moment we cannot tell everything but after the test reports are available, we can.

Mrs. XYZ: Can you tell me why do we get this discharge and will it affect my pregnancy?

Yes Mrs. XYZ, I can tell you about it.

The discharge could be normal or abnormal. Normally, most of the women get this colourless and odourless discharge. However, there are conditions like candidiasis, trichomoniasis, etc. which causes foul smelling discharge. All those occur in a condition called PID, i.e. pelvic inflammatory disease wherein there is infection of the reproductive organs. If found earlier then these can be treated by medications. But, if they reach a stage where it cannot be treated, then problem arises when they can damage the tube, womb, etc. and can harm reproduction.

In a good number of cases, the infections like gonorrhoea, etc. can occur or can be transmitted from the male partner and hence its important to run tests on both. The male not necessarily will exhibit the symptoms of the disease.

It is very important that both undergo the tests and also treatment. Meanwhile, practice safe sex, your partner should use condoms, avoiding multiple partners is good.

Is there anything else that you would like to know?

Thank you. I will provide you with necessary leaflets. You can go through them. Take care. Bye.

7. COUNSEL REGARDING STD

Hello, Mrs. XYZ, how are you feeling? I am Dr. ABC, Senior House Officer in Genitourinary Medicine. Well, before proceeding, I would like to assure you that whatever we are going to speak would be confidential. Now, may I know your concerns?

Mrs. ABC: I am worried I may be having STD as my husband had visited a prostitute. I am worried and want to know about STD and what will be done here.

Well, Mrs. XYZ, when was it and was it unprotected intercourse?

I understand your worries. STD is a disease that is transmitted through sexual intercourse. They could be the commoner ones like trichomoniasis, herpes, gonorrhoea and uncommon ones like HIV and syphilis.

I would like to ask you a few questions Mrs. XYZ

◆ Did you notice any discharge in your front passage?

◆ Do you have any soreness or itching down below?

◆ Any wound or ulcers? Do you have burning waterworks?

◆ Did you notice any changes in private parts of your partner like ulcer, soreness, any sweating?

These are the common features that can occur following an infection. Now, what we will do here is –

◆ Examine you thoroughly

◆ Test of water sample

◆ Blood test for routine investigations

◆ Blood test for HIV, syphilis

◆ Test of any discharge, if there is

◆ Test for the organisms if present

◆ TV scan of your tummy

Few reports will be given back on the same day, while others will take some time. We will give the necessary medications accordingly. Do not worry; we are there to take care of you. Bye.

8. COUNSEL REGARDING AIDS

A young male Mr Daniel, wants to get HIV test done following unprotected intercourse with an unknown lady. He is worried that he might have AIDS.

Hello, I am Dr. ABC. How are you Mr. Daniel? As far as I know you have come here to undergo HIV test. Before I proceed I assure you that it is going to be confidential. Now, can you tell me why you want to get this test done? Can you tell me whatever you know about this AIDS?

Yes, that is right.

HIV is the virus that causes AIDS and if a person is infected by this virus it does not mean that he had AIDS, it takes around 10-15 years for one to develop AIDS after HIV. By doing the test, there are many legal matters that you must bear in mind.

1. The HIV status can be asked during job offers when you will be bound to tell.

2. Insurance, mortgages may be denied sometimes.

3. It is important that you inform your partner/partners and your GP should be informed.

The test will be done at least three times. If we do it now, there are high chances of the test being negative, as during first 3 months of the infection, the virus may not show itself. So, we need to repeat it.

If the test is positive, we need to repeat it again to confirm it.

It is very important to note that you will be offered medications against HIV (initial stage) and against other infections that are common during HIV status positive. Take care –

1. Not to donate blood.

2. Better to avoid intercourse or at least use condoms. Inform your partner.

3. Avoid drugs as much as possible.

Anyway, we will take one step at a time now. Is there anything else that you want to know? Thanks.

9. BLOOD TRANSFUSION (JEHOVAH'S WITNESS)

Hello, I am Dr. ABC, Senior House Officer in Medicine. How are you feeling Mrs. Penny? May I know why you have been refusing blood transfusion?

Mrs. Penny: Because I am Jehovah's witness.

Dr. ABC: Well, I do respect your views and I cannot force you, but then, are you aware of how important it is to undergo blood transfusion?

If it is less amount of blood that is lost during the surgery then we can compensate by using fluids, but if larger amount is lost as in major surgery, then we can replace this only by giving blood so that –

◆ You will feel better

◆ Recover faster

◆ Body will respond positively

The blood is being collected from healthy volunteers after we take relevant history, examine them and also carry on with tests. We maintain high standards and thus prevent the chance of infection such as malaria, HIV, hepatitis-B.

Well, thinking of the benefits and in terms of your health, what we would advise is to get a transfusion if the need arises.

But then as I said earlier, you have the rights to refuse and seek a second opinion as well. I need to document this and would be glad if you could read it and then sign it.

If you would like to consult my senior colleague, then you can, I will arrange it for you.

Is there anything else? Take care and thanks for listening so patiently.

10. TESTICULAR TUMOUR

Hello, I am Dr. ABC, Senior House Officer in Surgery. How are you feeling Mr. Tomkins? Well, may I know your concerns? I can understand your worries. As my colleague has already spoken to you, we have found that there is a lump in your testis. I cannot tell you the exact diagnosis now, as we need to run a few tests.

The tumour or lump could be benign, i.e. harmless or cancerous. But, as I already said, we cannot comment on the diagnosis. We will do the following tests —

◆ Blood tests and will find out if certain hormones/chemicals that are raised or if normal
◆ We will **definitely not collect** sample of cells from the tumour as in other cases where we do because this can result in spreading of the tumour further.
◆ Also, we will do special TV scan also.

Do you have anything else to ask?

Mr. Tomkins: What if its cancer?
Well, if it is cancer, then a surgery will be done to remove the tumour with the testis on the affected side.

I can understand that you may be worried about fertility after removal of the testis, but you can become a father with the other testis. Its also seen that maximum number of people with cancer of testis have good prognosis after the surgery.

Is there anything else that you would like to know? I will be glad to answer you. Take care and thanks for listening patiently.

11. GONORRHOEA—CONTACT TRACING

Hello, Mr. Carneen, I am Dr. ABC, Senior House Officer in Genitourinary Medicine, i.e. GUM clinic. How are you? Before I can proceed I would like to mention that whatever we are going to discuss would be confidential and private.

As you know you came to us with problems in your waterworks and after examining you and running a few tests we have come to a conclusion that it is due to gonorrhoea. Do you know anything about it?

It is an infection due to unprotected sexual intercourse, which you said you had, and we did make a note of it during our last consultation.

We will give you a course of antibiotics and you should not have intercourse until you have been cured fully.

But more important is a few answers which I need from you. I know that these questions will be unpleasant to answer but they are very important to diagnose your problem.

◆ Do you have a stable partner?

◆ Can you tell me your sexual preference? (I mean which sex and which route) We want to treat your partner at the same time as you.

Mr. Carmeen, your partner may be having this infection or may get it and you may get re-infected. This disease will just continue to spread if we do not treat it. I know that it is private information, but I am duty bound to ask you that I need to talk to your partner as well.

I very well know that I cannot force you; I will note this refusal in the record, as I have to document this for legal purposes. You can seek my senior's advice if you are willing to. (If the patient refuses to reveal).

Is there anything else that you would like to know?
Take care and thanks.

12. MANAGING ANKLE INJURY

Hello, Mr. John, I am Dr. ABC, Senior House Officer in Orthopaedics. How are you feeling? How is the pain in your leg now? Well, I am here to talk to you about the management.

◆ **P**—First of all, we will give you the necessary **painkillers**, initially PCT, later NSAIDs if needed.

◆ **R**—You need to **rest** your foot, keep it elevated, and place two pillows below your feet while lying down.

◆ **I**—You can apply frozen peas or **ice cubes** over the ankle to reduce the swelling and pain. Keep it not for more than 7-10 minutes at a time.

◆ **C**—There are elastic bandages or tubi-grips or **crepe bandages** available which we will teach how to use. Remember that it should not be very tight, or too loose; remove it before going to sleep.

◆ **E**—**Exercise** your leg and ankle, so that the muscles do not waste but become stronger.

◆ Wriggle your toes.

◆ Move your foot up and down and round and round at the ankle.
This will strengthen the muscles.

◆ You can bear weight on injured foot only as much as you feel comfortable with.

◆ If you feel the swelling increases or if pain increases, contact your GP immediately or come to the A+E.

I hope this is not too much for you.
Do you have any queries? Thank you and take care.

13. ECZEMA

Mrs. Germy creek has come with her 25-year-old daughter complaining of itching and white rashes on her body that was diagnosed as eczema. Counsel her regarding this and answer her queries.

Hello I am Dr. X, Senior House Officer in Dermatology. How are you feeling today Mrs. Germy? How are you feeling Miss Grey? As you know you have been troubled a lot due to this rash and itch since a long-time. We examined you thoroughly and ran few tests as well and have found out that its eczema. Do you know anything about it? I am here to explain you every thing in detail and also to answer all your questions about it. If you are not able to follow you can stop me at any moment. Is that OK?

What is eczema?
It is a condition of the skin occurring due to the body reacting abnormally to certain substances, but this reaction does not occur in a person normally.
This basically causes the itching and peeling of skin and rashes as well. Sometimes it can become painful due to the persistent itching.

Will this ever reduce at all?
There are chances of this condition to reduce gradually, though the exact time is not known.

Why did this start? What could be the cause?

Actually most of the time the exact cause is not known, as I said it is an allergy and could be brought about by anything below the sun such as pets, flowers, gardening, woollen clothes, nylon material, feathers, soap, hot water.

It is also known to run in families.

Can something be done about it?

Of course yes.

◆ Avoid dust, pollen, pets, any irritant cream or soap. Avoid food that you are allergic to. Use warm water rather than the hot one.

◆ Clean your house regularly.

◆ Vacuum the sofa set and also duvet and pillows including the curtains.

◆ We will also provide you medications in the form of a cream, which contains steroid. You can use it over the sites where there are these rashes. Use it regularly everyday.

◆ You can also use moisturizer as and when needed.

Steroids I heard can be harmful?

It is only the long-term usage of steroid that will be harmful as causing increased weight, thinning of the skin and bones, irregular periods. There are also chances of infection as the immunity may fall.

It is not that all the people using steroid get these but I am duty bound to explain this as well.

Is there anything else that you would like to know?

I would be glad to help you.

I will provide you with the necessary leaflets and information sheets and also the details of **National Eczema Society** that you can go through it.

I appreciate your co-operation. Take care, bye.

14. ALZHEIMER'S DISEASE

Mr. Rich is admitted with behaving strangely since a few months and following examination he was diagnosed as having Alzheimer's disease, his daughter Miss. Jolie is anxious about it. Counsel her.

Hello I am Dr. ABC, Senior House Officer in Psychiatry. How are you feeling today Miss. Jolie?

As you know your father has been troubled with forgetfulness and behaving in a strange manner since a few days. We examined him thoroughly and ran few tests as well and have found out that its Alzheimer's disease.

Do you know anything about it? I am here to explain you everything in detail and also to answer all your questions about it. If you are not able to follow you can stop me at any moment. Is that OK?

What is this disease?
It is an illness affecting the memory causing dementia and over a period of time it would reduce the ability to reason and also concentrate.

This was what I feared. What he is going through is hurting all of us?
I can understand that Miss Jolie.

Well is he in the terminal stages or is this the beginning?
This is the beginning and there are chances that the condition may remain as it is or worsen further.

So what actually is the cause for this?
Most of the time we do not have the exact cause for this condition, but then its noted that it runs in the family, could be due to a viral infection.
Ultimately the brain shrinks to a smaller size due to accumulation of certain substances.

Now what are the problems that we can expect from this dementia?
◆ People with Alzheimer's forget place, people, time, situation and surrounding. They may not be able to recognize their loved ones.
◆ They will wander away from home as they forget places.
◆ They will not be bothered about their food habits and dressing as well. They may remain unkempt.
◆ They may pee or poo in any place.
◆ They may get irritated and start fighting as well.

Can't I do any thing to help my father?
I appreciate this Miss Jolie there are so many things that can be done like:
◆ Can keep away all sharp things away.
◆ Keep important documents and valuable things locked.
◆ Remove the locks from his room and also from the bathroom.

PLAB-2

◆ Keep a reminder for him and ask him to read it so that he does not forget things or he can have the talking reminder.

◆ Since these people are known to get irritated and agitated you have to be calm accepting his illness.

◆ Since this is a tedious job, you can always accept help from the social services, from your family and friends.

We here will work as a multidisciplinary team involving all the other departments and offer the services of a community nurse, occupational therapist and physio-therapist as well.

Psychiatrist also will be involved.

Both of you can avail your allowances. Your father can avail disability allowance and you the carer allowance.

I can understand that all this is very stressful, but then we are trying to help you as much as possible.

You need to relax and take a break sometimes as well. Look after your health as well.

Is there anything else that you would like to know?

I would be glad to help you.

I will provide you with the necessary leaflets and information sheets and also the details of Alzheimer's Disease Society that you can go through.

I appreciate your co-operation. Take care, bye.

15. SCHIZOPHRENIA

Mr. Halle has come to the Psychiatry department with his son being diagnosed as Schizophrenic. He wants to talk to you about it.

Hello, I am Dr. X, Senior House Officer in Psychiatry. How are you feeling today Mr. Halle?

As you know you got your son here with few problems, we examined him thoroughly and I am afraid the news is not good.

He is diagnosed as suffering from Schizophrenia. Do you know anything about it?

I am here to explain you every thing in detail and also to answer all your questions about it. If you are not able to follow you can stop me at any moment. Is that OK?

I have heard that it is a mental illness and here its 2-5 different people reside in a single body isn't it?

This is not split personality disorder that you are thinking of. It is schizophrenia, a common condition.

Here he will feel as if he is a zombie or a robot and that someone or some supernatural power is controlling him totally. He may feel as if his thoughts are being stolen from his mind or someone is putting thoughts into his mind. He may even feel that someone is watching him and all his movements recorded.

Sometimes they may even feel that some plot is being planned against them. They may lose interest in life. Feel hopeless and worthless. They may be totally cut off from this world and may not respond to any kind of emotions.

Why should he suffer with this?

Most of the time we don't have an exact cause for this, but its known to run in families, could be due to difficult delivery or even a viral infection. It is also caused due to the use of recreational drugs.

Is there anything that can be done?

Yes of course.

It is very important that he stays back here in the hospital, as the initial part of the treatment is very important.

◆ We will start off with medications. Apart from this, we will also provide
◆ The services of a community nurse
◆ Help him with his schooling
◆ Day care
◆ Employment help
◆ Recreation
◆ Rehabilitation

Is there any chance of him recovering?

Now, this depends on how the treatment goes on and how he responds to the treatment. Studies have shown that one-third of the patients recover, while one-third cases goes to become lifelong and in another one-third of them the condition or the illness recurs after treatment.

Is there anything else that you would like to know?

I will provide you with the details of —
1. **National Schizophrenia Fellowship (NSF)**
2. **SANELINE**
3. **MIND**

These are a few organizations from where you can seek help and information as well. They provide support and also help.

Is there anything else that you would like to know?

I would be glad to help you.

I will provide you with the necessary leaflets and information sheets.

I appreciate your co-operation. Take care, bye.

16. HARMFUL EFFECTS OF ALCOHOL

Counsel regarding the harmful effects of alcoholism to Mr. Collin who was admitted following vomiting blood and severe gastritis.

Hello, Mr. Collin. I am Dr. X, Senior House Officer in Medicine. How are you feeling today? I am glad that you have recovered well. I would like to have a small chat with you. Is that OK with you?

As you know that all these problems arised due to the drinks, which I am sure you are aware of by now.

Drinking in moderate amounts will not harm in this way as how it does by drinking more than the safety limit.

Are you aware of the problems that drinks can cause?
1. First of all the problems with which you presented will increase and you may suffer from severe gastritis.
2. It can damage any and every organ in the body.
3. It can cause ulcer formation in the lips, mouth, throat, food pipe, stomach and the bowel or in severe cases cancer of these parts.
4. It is also known to cause blood loss in the form of vomiting blood or as passing blood through the poo.
5. It also causes a raise in the blood pressure.
6. It can affect the brain and reduces the capacity to understand a situation.
7. It affects the liver and can cause decrease in the size of the liver.
8. Can also affect the libido.

9. The major harm that it can cause is in the family and also affects social life. This may therefore cause financial problems, unnecessary fights.

10. You may get in trouble with the law.

11. Drinking and driving can also prove to be dangerous both to you and the others.

12. Liver failure can also occur.

13. This also can affect your work.

These are just a few of the problems that can occur.

All that I would like to tell is that the benefits of giving up drinking is more than anything else.

This will be tough initially but with strong determination and will power anything is possible.

We are there to help you regarding this matter.

Right now I will provide you with the leaflets and important information sheets that will be helpful and we will talk about it later.

Do you have any questions to ask?

How can you help me?
◆ By giving medicines which will help in quitting this habit.
◆ Self-help groups.
◆ Services of health care workers and the community nurses.
◆ Rehabilitation programmes.

It is ultimately again in your hands. From our side you will have strong support.

I appreciate your co-operation. Take care, bye.

17. CHRONIC FATIGUE SYNDROME

Mr. Rigbert has come to the clinic with feeling tired since around 7 months and it is recurring once every few days. The condition has been diagnosed as Chronic Fatigue Syndrome. Counsel him regarding this and about the management also.

Hello, I am Dr.X, Senior House Officer in Medicine. How are you feeling today Mr. Rigbert?

As you know you had come to us with feeling tired since a few months and we examined you thoroughly and after running few tests we have diagnosed it as chronic fatigue syndrome (CFS). Do you know anything about it?

I am here to explain you everything in detail and also to answer all your questions about it. If you are not able to follow you can stop me at any moment. Is that OK?

What is this illness?

It is a condition where in the person feels tired and gets fatigued easily even on doing normal work and this happens without him straining as well.

But how does this start? I have always been a healthy person, except the common cold I have never had any other problems at all.

In most of the cases the CFS starts following a cold or lung infection, or infection of the liver- hepatitis or due to tummy problems. In few of them it could be due to viral infection. Stress can also cause this sometimes.

Can you tell me something more about his CFS?

Sure.

◆ Usually the person suffers from fatigue for more than 6 months without any cause.

They may have the following conditions as well along:

Throat pain

Muscle pain

Headache

Joint pain

Painful glands in the body.

Sleep, which is unsatisfactory.

Depression

And to actually inform I had a cold and headache as well. Now, can anything be done for this?

Actually, there is no permanent cure for this condition; we can however correct the different problems individually. This will be very helpful.

The first phase of treatment includes:

1. Taking steps to reduce stress.

2. To help you in identifying the cause for disturbed sleep and then try for stress free and restful sleep.

3. Relieving the various pains by simple painkillers and heat packs.

4. Relieving bone/joint pain and stiffness with medicines such as Ibuprofen.

5. To help you sleep better and for the depression we can give TCA and another medicine that is SSRI.

6. To find out what the triggering factor is and preventing it.

Will this detiorate further?

Well we cannot tell how it will proceed, but we will try to help you as much as possible. Moreover it is not a progressive condition and it causes no permanent damage.

We will try the medicines and see how well your body is going to respond. It may be necessary to change the medicine and sometimes to change the dosage as well or to try a different approach.

All this will be basically to find out which mode of treatment will suit you the best. We will also provide counselling sessions for you and your family.

Is there anything else that you want to know about?

I will provide you with the leaflets, website address, self-help group address.

They will be very helpful, we will have regular follow-ups.

You have been very co-operative.

Thanks, take care.

18. JAUNDICE IN NEWBORN BABY

Hello, I am Dr. X. I am Senior House Officer in Paediatrics. How are you feeling now Mrs. Jones? Congratulations for the cute baby boy you have delivered.

Well he have examined him thoroughly and have noticed that he is having a condition called jaundice, it is not a disease. Do you know about it?

Liver is an organ in our tummy and this regulates a certain chemical called bile in our body. Sometimes this chemical increases so much that it cannot be broken or regulated in the liver and instead increases in our body. This causes yellowing of skin, eyes the water and also waste.

Is it dangerous?

If the level of chemical increases it can reach the brain and affect the brain.

Is there any treatment available?

Well there are, but before that we need to run further tests on his water and blood. There are different methods available.

1. Exchange transfusion:

    Here we will give warm blood into his vein and remove the blood from his body.

2. We will give antibiotics if its due to infection.

3. Phototherapy:

    Here we will focus light from special source. This is the method we follow during starting stages, that is when the chemical is not so very high.

This can result in loss of some amount of salts in his body but we will take care of that also.

But why my little one?

◆ It could be due to difference in blood group between your little one and you.

◆ Infections also can cause it.

Is there anything else you would like to know?

I appreciate your co-operation. I will come back to you again. Take care.

19. IRRITABLE HIP SYNDROME

Hello, Mrs. Keith, how are you feeling. I am Dr. X, Senior House Officer in Orthopaedics. As far as I know you had come to us with little Johan having hip joint pain. I am here to have a small talk regarding this, is that OK? If you are not able to follow, you can stop me at any moment. After examining him and also taking an X-ray we have found out that there is no disease of the joint. This condition is called Irritable hip syndrome.

Do you know anything about it?

Why does this occur?

It is a common condition seen in boys of age group 3-8 years where in they present with pain in the hip and difficulty in moving the leg for sometime.

This is not a dangerous condition at all and not life-threatening at all.

As the age increases the condition subsides and disappears.

It is basically the inflamation of the hip joint, there is irritation of the hip and hence the name.

This pain if severe we will give painkillers and he has to resume with his movements slowly during the time he has pain. He needs to take rest during that time.

There is nothing to worry about, we will have regular follow-up here. We will perform X-rays and blood tests also.

Is there anything else that you want to know?

I appreciate your co-operation.

I will provide you with the leaflets and information sheet, you can go through them. Do not worry we will take care of him.

Take care and bye.

11 Calculation

I. CALCULATE THE NORMAL SALINE NEEDED

1. In a child weighing 4 kgs, midazolam needed as dose of 4 µg/kg/hr at a rate of 3 ml/hr for 1 day. [1 ml of midazolam = 1mg]. Calculate the normal saline needed for dilution.

Solution

Weight = 4 kg

Rate = 3 ml/hr

Dose = 4 µg/kg/hr

1 ml = 1 mg

(a) Total fluid needed is 3 ml for 1 hours

∴Total fluid needed for 24 hours

= 3 × 24 = 72 ml

(b) Dose of Midazolam

4 µg/kg/hr

∴ 4 µg × 4 kgs × 24 hr

Total dose = 4 × 4 × 24 = 384 µg = 0.384 mg

(c) 1 mg = 1 ml of midazolam

∴ 0.384 mg = ? = 0.384 ml of midazolam

(d) 72 ml of fluid contains 0.384 ml of midazolam

∴ The normal saline is 72-0.384 ml

= 71.616 ml

Ans = 71.616 ml of NS

I will confirm it however with a senior and will ensure that the medicine has not passed its expiry date.

2. **In a baby of 4 kg who needs 25 µg/kg/hr of morphine at a rate of 1 ml/hr; 1 ml amp = 1 mg. Calculate the normal saline needed for dilution for one day.**

   Weight = 4 kg
   Rate = 1 ml/hr
   Dose = 25 µg/kg/hr
   1 ml = 1 mg
(a) Total fluid = 1 ml/hr
   ∴ For 1 day = 24 × 1 = 24 ml
(b) Dose = 25 µg/kg/hr
        = 25 µg × 4 ×24 = 2400 µg = 2.4 mg
(c) 1 mg = 1 ml of morphine
   ∴ 2.4 mg = ?
   2.4 ml
(d) Total fluid is 24 ml
   ∴ NS is 24-2.4 = 21.6 ml
   Ans = 21.6 ml of NS

I will confirm the findings with my senior and will ensure that I am not using medicine that has passed beyond expiry date.

3. **In an adult of 40 kg who needs midazolam at a rate of 1 ml/hr at a dose of 20 µg/kg/hr for 1 day[1 ml amp = 1 mg], calculate the normal saline needed.**

   Weight = 40 kg
   Rate = 1 ml/hr
   Dose = 20 µg/kg/hr
   1 ml = 1 mg
(a) Total fluid = 1 × 24 = 24 ml
(b) Total dose = 20 µg/kg/hr
        = 20 × 40 × 24   = 19200 µg
                              = 19.2 µg
(c) 1 mg = 1 ml of midazolam
   19.2 mg = ?   → 19.2 ml
(d) 24 ml of fluid contains 19.2 ml of midazolam.
   So, NS is 24 – 19.2 = 4.8 ml
   Ans = 4.8 ml of NS

I will confirm the findings with my senior and will ensure that I am not using medicine that has passed beyond expiry date.

II. TO CALCULATE THE RATE AT WHICH THE MEDICINE HAS TO BE GIVEN

1. Calculate the total dose and the rate at which morphine has to be given to a child weighing 3 kg, at a dose of 20 µg/kg/hr and 1 ml amp = 10 mg of morphine. Use NS for dilution.

Solution:

Weight = 3 kg

Dose = 20 µg/kg/hr

1 ml = 10 mg

(a) Total dose = 20 µg/kg/hr

   = 20 × 3 = 60 µg/hr

(b) 1 amp = 1 ml = 10 mg

1 ml = 10000 µg

∴ 0.6 ml = 6000 µg

(c) Take 0.6 ml of morphine and add to 99.4 ml of NS to make it 100 ml.

100 ml solution = 99.4 ml (NS) + 0.6 ml (Mor)

100 ml has 0.6 ml

100 ml has 6000 µg

∴ 1 ml has? →60 mg

We are giving the medicine as 60 mg/hr but 60 mg = 1 ml

∴ 1 ml/ hr

Ans: The rate at which morphine has to be given as 1 ml/hr.

III. TO PREPARE INSULIN INFUSION

Prepare 500 ml infusion @ 1U/hr in 100 ml (1 ml insulin = 100 units)

Solution:

(a) Take 1 ml of insulin (100 U) and add 9 ml of NS.

(b) 10 ml of fluid = 1ml = 100 U

   10 ml of fluid = 100 U

   1 ml fluid = 10 U

   0.5 ml fluid = 5 U

(c) Add 499.5 ml of NS to 0.5 ml of fluid so 500 ml of fluid has 5 U of insulin. Thus 100 ml has 1 U/hr i.e., 100 ml which has 1 U insulin per hour.

Ans: 500 ml infusion can be given as simply as 1 U/hr, i.e. in 100 ml/hr.

HOW TO COLLECT ON A SYRINGE

(a) 100 U/ml is available.

(b) 5 U is needed [i.e., $\dfrac{100\ U}{0.05\ ml} = \dfrac{0.01\ U/ml]}{ml}$ (100 U = 1 ml

   5 U = ? = 0.05 ml)

(c) Take 4 units on syringe, it implies 0.04 ml. Put it into the saline bag.

(d) Now take 2 units in the syringe, i.e., 0.02 ml and dilute it to the mark of 4 units so we have 0.04 ml (that is diluted). Take half of this i.e., 0.02 ml which since diluted is equal to 1 u only so install this into the saline bag. Thus, 5 units installed.

PLAB-2

Recent Examination Papers

SEPTEMBER-8-2004

1. Counsel a mother who has brought her child with incessant crying since 1 week
2. Suturing
3. Myocardial infarction—viva
4. Counsel a young lady with eczema
5. Pervaginal examination
6. Lady with MCV posted for toe nail removal surgery. Ellicit history of alcoholism.
7. CPR
8. ABG analysis
9. Otoscopy
10. History of loss of consciousness
11. Diabetic foot examination
12. History of tiredness and bodyache for 6 months (CFS)
13. Counsel mother about her child having diarrhoea (telephone conversation)
14. Counsel regarding ectopic pregnancy

SEPTEMBER-14-2004

1. History of palpitation.
2. History of pain abdomen.
3. Otoscopy.
4. I.V cannulation.
5. Examination of cranial nerves II-VII.
6. Viva—DKA.
7. Examination of knee.
8. CPR.

9. History of breathlessness.
10. Depression- History and counselling.
11. Counsel regarding epilepsy.
12. Counsel about pain management in labour.
13. Counsel about ovarian cystectomy.
14. BP measurement.

SEPTEMBER-27-2004

1. Urinary catheterization.
2. Ellicit history of alcoholism.
3. Primary survey.
4. Examination of knee.
5. Counselling about ectopic pregnancy.
6. History of haematuria.
7. Examination of knee.
8. Counselling about epilepsy.
9. CPR.
10. PEFR.
11. I.V cannulation.
12. Thyroid examination.
13. History of severe headache.

OCTOBER-21-2004

1. Examination of wrist.
2. Pervaginal examination.
3. History of joint pain.
4. CPR.
5. Suturing.
6. ABG.
7. Examination of diabetic foot.
8. Counsel regarding appendicectomy.
9. History of haematuria.
10. Telephone conversation with registrar about intestinal obstruction.

PLAB-2

11. Counsel regarding medications for asthma and use of inhalers.
12. History taking from a mother with a baby who had sustained fracture femur and multiple bruises.
13. Counsel regarding HIV test.
14. Patient with lack of sleep, counsel her.

OCTOBER-27-2004

1. CPR.
2. Secondary survey.
3. History of fever.
4. Counselling – herniorrhaphy and pain relief.
5. History of childabuse.
6. Dose calculation of insulin
7. Respiratory system examination.
8. Counselling ectopic pregnancy.
9. Urinary catheterization.
10. Counselling appendicectomy.
11. Per rectal examination.
12. Blood pressure measurement.
13. History of weight loss.
14. Examination of wrist joint.

NOVEMBER-2-2004

1. Respiratory examination and PEFR.
2. CPR.
3. Diabetic foot examination.
4. Dose calculation of insulin.
5. History of headache.
6. History of dysphagia.
7. Otoscopy.
8. BP.
9. Counselling–Irritable hip syndrome.
10. Catheterization.

11. MMSE.
12. Counselling–Nephrectomy.
13. History of childabuse.
14. History of amenorrhoea.

NOVEMBER-9-2004

1. BP
2. Neurological examination of lower limbs (diabetic patient).
3. Counselling – Post MI medication.
4. Assess risk factor for stroke.
5. History of weight loss in 16-year-old girl.
6. Cervical smear.
7. Counselling about mesothelioma.
8. Examination of elbow.
9. Examination of upper abdomen.
10. History of haematuria.
11. Counsel about ovarian cystectomy.
12. Counsel mother about her son who had met with RTA and needs spleenectomy and Rx for fracture femur.
13. I.V cannulation.
14. CPR.

DECEMBER-10-2004

1. Thyroid examination
2. Venepuncture
3. Suturing
4. BP measurement
5. CPR—Paediatric
6. MMSE
7. History and counselling—Osteoporosis
8. Counselling—Herniorrhaphy
9. Per vaginal examination
10. History of polydipsia in lethargic child—History taking

11. History taking—Obesity
12. Examination—Peripheral vascular disease
13. Epilepsy—Counselling regarding life style changes
14. Telephone conversation—Intestinal obstruction

DECEMBER-13-2004

1. Catheterization
2. Pervaginal examination
3. Venepuncture
4. CPR—Paediatric
5. Primary survey
6. Asthma—Counselling
7. Peripheral vascular disease—Examination
8. Counselling—Drug abuse
9. Counselling—Epilepsy
10. Evaluate for day care surgery
11. Chest pain—History
12. Bleeding per rectum—History
13. BP
14. Counselling—Herniorrhaphy

JANUARY-12-2005

1. BP measurement
2. ABG—Blood sampling
3. CPR—Adult
4. Per rectal examination
5. Primary survey
6. Febrile convulsion—History
7. Ear pain—History
8. Haemoptysis—History
9. Counselling—Labour pain management
10. Counselling—Migraine
11. Counselling—Irritable hip syndrome

12. Counselling—Meningitis
13. Shoulder examination
14. PTSD—History

JANUARY-21-2005

1. CPR—Child
2. BP measurement
3. Cervical smear
4. Venepuncture
5. CVA—History taking
6. Cough + wheeze—History taking
7. RUQ pair—History taking
8. Counselling—Crying child
9. Counselling—PET
10. Counselling—Cancer prostate in terminal stages
11. Meningitis examination
12. Hip examination
13. MMSE

JANUARY-31-2005

1. Venepuncture
2. Catheterization
3. CPR—Paediatric
4. Breast examination
5. Thyroid examination
6. Counselling—Epilepsy
7. Herniorrhaphy—Counselling
8. Per vaginal examination
9. Diarrhoea in a child—History
10. Chest pain—History
11. DKA—Viva
12. BP—measurement
13. Counselling—Postnatal depression
14. Counselling—Rheumatoid hand

Index

PLAB-2

PLAB-2